To Dina,

Wishing you God's
best in every time of
your life.

B.C.

The Time
of Her Life

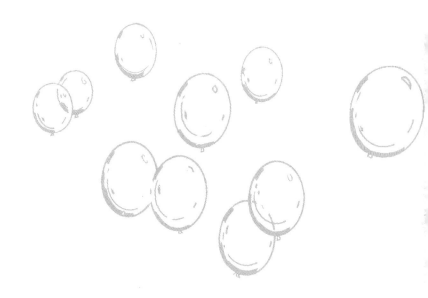

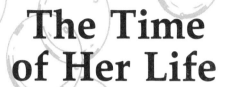

The Time
of Her Life

Meg Woodson

ZONDERVAN PUBLISHING HOUSE
of The Zondervan Corporation
Grand Rapids, Michigan

THE TIME OF HER LIFE
© 1982 by Meg Woodson

First printing, April 1982

Library of Congress Cataloging in Publication Data
Woodson, Meg.
      The time of her life.

            1. Woodson, Margaret Ann. 2. Woodson, Meg.
3. Christian biography — United States. 4. Cystic
fibrosis — Patients — United States — Biography. I.
Title.
BR1713.W645   248.8′6′0922 [B]   82-2747
ISBN 0-310-34870-6   AACR2

Edited by Judith E. Markham
Designed by Kim Koning

Printed in the United States of America

To Memphis Grandmother and Grandfather
And to New York Grandmother
And to New York Grandfather, who, since the
writing of this book, has gone to clap in
the highest mountains.

Contents

For their participation in the preparation of this book:

My thanks to my daughter, Peggie, who is the book, and to my husband, who cares more about the book and its author than anyone else.

My thanks also to the members of the Cuyahoga County Writers Workshop for giving their most valued possession, their own writing time, to read and evaluate my writing.

And to Philip Yancey, who answered my harried calls for help helpfully.

And to Anna Setar, who listened when I was discouraged.

And to Laura Yahner, who prays for my writing every day.

To the Reader

Three things I want you to know about the story in this book.

The first is that the story is true. So much cover-up covers up the world today, that we long for truth. We still find magic in make-believe, but a greater magic in *once upon a real time*. So while I have changed names in my story and often the chronology of events and other incidental factors, essentially I am telling you the story as Peg and I recorded it and remember it.

The second thing I want you to know is that I'm having a hard time telling the story. The quiet creaks through this huge, hollow house as I sit here at the dining room table surrounded by diaries and picture albums and date books and memory boxes reconstructing the past four and a half years of Peggie's life. Sometimes at night when I can't sleep for absorbing the hush of my emptied nest, I wander from bed to bed; and when I wake up in the morning, it takes me an unnerving moment to decide where I am. I don't know why I want you to know about the hard part; I just do.

The third and main thing I want you to know, though, is that the story you are about to read is a triumphant story. Not because tragic things don't happen in it, but because it is Peggie's story.

"You amaze me, mother," she told me once. "The way you stay angry or depressed for so long. Sometimes I try to be sad about something I think I should be sad about, but I can't make it last. Or I try to stay mad. I mean, you've never known it, but sometimes I've made up my mind I would not talk to you and father for a whole day. But I could never stick with it for more than an hour or two. It's like I have to be happy."

The story consists of a series of portraits of Peggie's journey through those bewitched, bedeviled adolescent years in which a young girl becomes a woman. I paint these portraits partly for teenagers and the parents of teenagers to help them know they are not alone in the conflicts which so disrupt this time of life, and to help ease those conflicts.

But more basically, I paint the portraits for all people who are waging a losing war with whatever stage of life they're in, with whatever their agonies and aspirations. For already with fledgling arms Peg has flailed her way through to more victories over herself and her society than most of us achieve in a lifetime.

A sad, defeated world needs to watch Peggie grow up.

I don't say this because she's perfect. Goodness knows, she berates her mother more than any mother deserves to be berated. Nor do I say it because she's my daughter. I say it because somewhere along the line Peg has given herself to Another, and Another has given Himself to Peg. And from that God-girl union has come the story of imperfect glory you are about to read.

Fourteen Years Old

Peg and I are shopping for her first bra—padded. "I don't feel right about it, mother," she keeps saying. "It doesn't seem honest."

Lerners doesn't have doors on its dressing rooms, and Peggie leads the way to the last cubicle so as few people as possible can look in. She tries on the first of our selections and stands there, arms stretched out to her sides, hands drooping. "You surely do not expect me to wear one of these contraptions for the rest of my life," she sputters.

And then a tiny cherub face haloed with amber ringlets appears under the partition that separates our cubicle from the next in line, and boy eyes gaze up at Peggie wonderingly. Peg glares down at the little innocent. "Go a-way!" she hisses. "GO A-WAY!"

The soft, brown eyes don't blink, but *go away* in such a flash Peg hoots with laughter. She hoots with such abandon that as soon as she stops, the mother in the next cubicle chuckles loudly, and as soon as the mother stops, the teenagers in the booth beyond that fall into a fit of giggling. And so it goes until Peggie's laughter bounces booth by booth down the entire row of dressing rooms.

Peggie's laughing, however, soon turns into coughing. Any physical effort she makes leads to red-in-the-face coughing. This time when the cherub from next door reappears, his mother jerks him back. Peggie has become a menace.

Peggie should never undress surrounded on three sides by mirrors. Just when her friends are filling out, her chest is sinking in. Only her ribs protrude, and no way can she hide from her skeleton arms, the worst trial of her life. I cannot bear to look at the youthful horror with which Peggie looks at herself.

"So okay," she growls. "Which one of these things do I have to buy? It's all your idea, ya know." We decide on the bra that seems least likely to get bashed in.

"Now don't go tellin' daddy about this," she warns. "I don't want anybody lookin' at me." She scrambles into her red and blue striped top. "Do I look fourteen, mother?"

How many times she has asked a similar question. Do I look twelve? Do I look thirteen? I do? Well, what would you know, mother?

I glance at her covertly. Large eyes, blue as the sky; pretty, pug-nosed face; golden hair hanging straight at that in-between length, pulling you into its aura. She is a teenager. Yet how child-small she looks. How sick-small that five foot, almost one inch, seventy-two pounds of Margaret Ann Woodson looks.

"Well," I tell her, "fourteen covers a pretty wide range—from young fourteen to old fourteen. I'd say you definitely look fourteen."

"Oh? Well, what would you know, mother?"

Peg parts and re-parts her hair, fastening it back on one side with a daisy barrette, combing and re-combing the bangs that must always just reach the black plastic frames of her glasses. "You can sit on the floor if you want," she tells me, sitting on dressing room floors being a thing I do on desperate occasions when our shopping sprees go on and on.

I'm not tired on this occasion, this being our first stop of the day, but something in Peg's voice constrains me. Soon she is on the floor beside me, and I realize that she is the one who can no longer stand. I cannot think about it.

We lean against the wall, sides touching in the tiny room, Peg twirling her bra round and round on her forefinger. "Joey would have made a slingshot out of it, wouldn't he, mother?"

"Yes, Peg. Joey would have made a slingshot out of it." It was the kind of thing Joey had been best at. In the same category as creeping downstairs at Peg's fourteenth birthday slumber party, the loose sole of his left pajama foot flapping as he picked his way over the prostrate forms on the family room floor and waved his Coast Guard flares in fiendish outer-space motions.

Could that have happened on March 12th, just four months ago?

Peg, of course, had risen from out the bedlam and chased Joey from her party, yelling, as she found occasion to yell every March 12th, that for twenty-nine days, till he had his birthday, she would be three years older than he. And Joey, of course, yelled back, while fleeing up the stairs, that she was not the boss of him.

Joey had teased Peggie, and Peggie had bossed Joey. Yet brother and sister had been closer than most, bound together by their love of books and their stamp collections and their cystic fibrosis.* Every year they both put one of the birthday cards they received with their ages on the front on the mantel, where the cards huddled side by side till the next year.

Well, Joey'd had his twelfth birthday on April 10th, and on July 9th, two weeks ago, he had his death day.

Shopping for a bra was supposed to make Peggie feel that her life was going on. Maybe, too, if she looked less different, she'd feel and act less different, and next year the voices of her guests wouldn't swirl around and over her at her own party. Maybe if she looked older when school started in the fall, Eugene would stop shouting, "If you're dying, Peggie Woodson, why don't you hurry up?"

"I don't wanna shop for any more clothes," Peg pants as she hoists herself up from the dressing room floor. "I just wanna go home."

*Cystic fibrosis is a hereditary disease affecting the mucus-secreting and sweat glands of the body. Normally mucus performs a valuable protective and lubricating function. In the C.F. patient it becomes thick and sticky, clogging and prohibiting the normal functions of the pancreas, intestines, salivary glands, and lungs. It produces malnutrition, diarrhea, abnormal sweating, and eventually fatal lung disease. Patients are treated with digestive enzymes and antibiotics, aerosols and therapy—a pounding and vibrating on the lungs in various positions to encourage the mucus to run out. The mean age of death for a C.F. patient is twenty.

As we leave the store, she shoves the bag with the bra in it into my hands. "It still doesn't seem honest, mother. I mean, what will God think?"

"Well, honey, I think God understands that girls with cystic fibrosis develop more slowly than their friends. And just as I'm sure He's glad you can take antibiotics to help your cough and enzymes to help your digestion, I'm sure He's glad you can buy a padded bra to help you look like you would look if you didn't have C.F."

Surely God agrees that it is time for Peggie's undershirts to go.

"Hey, yeah!" Peg exclaims. "That sounds pretty good. Wasn't that funny, mother, all the people laughing booth by booth like that? Will you let me be the one to tell father at supper tonight about all the people laughing?"

* * * * *

This is your first trip back since Joey died, isn't it, mother?" Peg asks in response to the heavy hush in the car as we approach the hospital area of Cleveland. Suddenly she is a tour guide, gesturing dramatically. "This is an historic occasion, ladies and gentlemen."

"Oh, Peggie."

"Well, I have to do something to cheer you up. You wanna count the interesting things we see between here and the hospital like we did when I was little?"

And then before I can answer, she chatters on. "Remember that time we admitted Joey to the hospital, and when the intern came to examine him, Joey was makin' frantic faces behind his back, and he was holding on to his pants, and he was whispering, 'Ask the doctor can I leave on my pants. I forgot my underpants!'"

But when finally we reach the fourth floor of Rainbow Babies and Childrens Hospital, even Peg is silent.

I am weak with memories, but peer as I do into every room, I cannot remember which is *Joey's room.* Does Peg remember? "Didn't we have a good time with Joey the night we came and took him to his sixth grade graduation?" I ask as she stops halfway down the hall and leans against the wall to rest—a wounded bird of a girl, threadlike legs trembling, tender breast rising and falling and rasping with a frantic rapidity.

I wish Joe were with us, but Joe is a minister, and Sunday morning is the one time he cannot get away.

As soon as I settle Peg in her four-bed ward, I track down Dr. Rathburn. "Peggie's acting just like Joey acted the last time we brought him in." I think my unthinkable fear out loud, so Dr. Rathburn will deny it.

"I know," he says. "Her x-ray score is just one point above where Joey's was when the bottom dropped out."

"But . . . I'm not ready for that. . . ."

"I'm not ready for that either," says Dr. Rathburn.

A technician from the blood lab is with Peggie when I get back to her. "How's your brother, Peg?" he sings out. "How's your brother, Peggie?"

Peggie hangs her head.

"What's the matter? You do have a brother, don't you?"

"Not any more I don't," Peg says in a tiny, tearful voice and hangs her head lower still.

"You see that girl over there in the corner bed?" she asks when the technician leaves, giving me the belligerent eye lest I challenge her movement up to dryer ground. "Well, her name is Lucy, and she keeps putting on her light for the nurses to give her oxygen, but the nurses won't answer her light 'cause they say she only needs the oxygen psychologically. So I'm gonna be the one to give her her oxygen. I mean, I don't care why she needs it. She still needs it.

"Do you think that could be my ministry when I get to the point when I'm in the hospital a lot? Helpin' people? A lot of times the little kids will do stuff for me they won't do for the nurses."

Joe arrives in the early afternoon, a withdrawn look about him.

"Will you bring me that set of Children's Classics on the second shelf of my small bookcase when you come again?" Peg asks him. "I know they're for little kids, but they were so boring when I was little. Actually, every classic I ever read was boring. I thought I'd read 'em again, try to figure out what's good about 'em, ya know? Ya know, father? Why aren't you talkin', father?"

Joe leaves after supper—after a prayer and a hug, of course —for an evening meeting, but it is time for lights out before I gather my things together.

"Just can't wait to get away from me, can you, mother?"

I don't want to leave, but the only time I've stayed overnight in the hospital was during the last three weeks of Joey's life, and I don't think it would be good for Peg's outlook for me to stay.

I drive home through the dark. But what about her black teeth? I think. Will Peg be able to bear her teeth so discolored by antibiotics now that she has no one to have black teeth with?

Suddenly the emotions I have controlled through this endless day turn violent and control me. I weep. I weep. I pull the car off the road and give myself over to weeping. For the son I have lost and for the daughter I may lose. Could Eugene be right? Would it be better for Peg to hurry up with her dying, get it over with while her earnest desire to please God is intact? Her insistence on meaning for whatever time she has? Her love of learning and her cheeriness and courage? Before the cruelty of her peers destroys her concern for people? Before the pressures of a not-so-pure world violate her almost other-worldly purity?

Oh, God, I love Peg so just as she is, so tall and whole in spirit. But can she stay that way in this bent, unholy world? Please let her live, God—but as *Peggie,* the essence of all that has always been Peggie.

* * * * *

You know how on Thursday Dr. Rathburn took all us C.F. kids who were in the hospital and drove us over to C.F. Camp? Well, when I walked in the Council Room, the whole place was suddenly so quiet it was like you could feel your heart beating. And then all the boys were sayin', 'Joey Woodson's sister. Joey Woodson's sister.' And they were all coming over to me and saying, 'We're sorry, Peggie. We're sorry.' I thought I was gonna cry in front of the whole camp. "Patti was there, but she was with somebody else," she says, referring to her best C.F. friend, with whom she has done everything at C.F. Camp since C.F. Camp began, and with whom she has shared a room for several hospitalizations. "They had pictures up of other years at camp. I mean, they were just for show, but they gave me the ones with Joey in them. I don't blame Patti for not payin' attention to me. If I'd been there all week without her, I'd of found somebody else too."

Everybody worries about how Peggie must be reacting to Joey's death, but Peggie is going to be all right because she doesn't hide her hurts. She doesn't boast about them, but she doesn't bury them either.

She drags her precious collection of Casper and Richie Rich comic books into the middle of her bedroom floor. "I'm gonna get rid of these dumb comic books," she announces. "I only ever wanted them so I'd have more than Joey. Oh, mother, I don't have anybody any more to have more of anything than." Peggie pinpoints her particular hurts.

She comes back from playing up the street with Mary, Mary with the fighting brothers and sisters. "Oh, mother, you can't imagine how good it was to be in a house with noise." Peggie chokes on her own persistent perception.

Society has not yet programed her to restrain her tears. "I hate to go into Joey's room," she confides, "'cause every time I do, it's like he ought to be in there workin' on one of his three-thousand-piece puzzles. Ya know, with that brown hair of his all mussed up, and his glasses hanging over the sides of his ears instead of over the tops? I mean, every time I go in Joey's room, I cry. But then when I come out, I feel better."

The little kids in Sunday school were asking the teacher about dogs in heaven, and she was tellin' them about immortal souls and all. I told 'em heaven was a perfect place, and if they needed their dogs to be perfectly happy in heaven, their dogs would be there. I don't know why grownups make things so complicated." Peg has been an assistant teacher in Sunday school for several months now.

"Even you, mother. You're always wonderin' what heaven is like and what Joey is doing. Well, I saw a picture once of a little boy playing outside this big, golden palace, and that's the way I think of Joey. I mean, I know that's not the way he is, but since I don't know the way he is, that's the way I think of him—like he's doin' a ten-thousand-piece puzzle with an angel sorting.

"And you always want to know does Joey think about us, and how could he be perfectly happy if he knows what's going on down here. But I think God can fix things like that up. If Joey knows what's goin' on down here, God can fix it up so he can know but not feel bad. I don't know how He can do it, but I know He can do it.

"Why do grownups ask so many questions? Don't you want to be satisfied?"

Peggie is not without fear of death. "Does it hurt to die of cystic fibrosis?" she probes. She's afraid of the mechanics of death, and she's afraid of it because it's a new experience. "When my time comes, I'm not gonna be all calm and peaceful the way Joey was. When my time comes, you're gonna have to hire me a psychiatrist."

But concerning heaven, that golden-palace land to which death is the gate, Peggie has no fears. Nor does she falter unduly in relinquishing Joey to it. "Oh, father, how m-a-c-a-b-r-e," she spells a dozen times a day, impatient with what she considers the morbid, unrealistic aspects of Joe's and my grief. "Don't tell me you're gonna leave Joey's twelve-year-old card on the mantle. You are? Oh, mother, how m-a-c-a-b-r-e."

I have a hard time making myself clean out Joey's drawers. How can I do away forever with that joyous Joey-jumble of matchbox cars and model paints and clean and dirty socks? "You might as well do it, mother," Peg advises. "He's not gonna reappear by magic, ya know."

I get flowers and water ready to take to the cemetery. "I don't understand why you do that, mother. What are the flowers for? Oh, I get it. It's so things will look nice for people drivin' through." It's not that Peggie has no feelings; she just has no feeling that Joey is down there underneath the flowers.

She follows me out to the car. "I guess it's okay if you go, mama, as long as you know in your head he's not down there. One of these days it'll get down into your heart."

* * * * *

There's no point in your crying out in front of me," Peg reprimands me. "I tell you my common sense, but you won't listen. Joey turned out good, didn't he? How could he turn out so good if you were so bad? So why do you keep asking were you a good mother?"

"Joey and I spent a lot of time working on his monster models before he got sick," Joe worries. "Do you think the strong odor of the glue had anything to do with what happened in his lungs?"

"Oh, daddy, you always have a guilty conscience that makes you think ridiculous things. I mean, whenever anything good happens, you say God did it, but when anything bad happens, you say you did it. That's dumb. Are you payin' attention to me, father?

"I sure was awful to Joey," she admits of her own relationship to him. "Ya know how he would have one week to pick television programs and I would have the next? Well, I used to figure way ahead to when there would be a vacation week and count back and fix it so I'd get to pick then. I was terrible to him."

She thinks for a minute. "Just like a regular sister.

"And when we were in the hospital together the time before last, and the nurses made him walk up and down the hall seven times? I mean, nobody would listen when he said how tired he was. And he came in my room in that 'itty bitty wheelchair all exhausted and tried to tell me about it, and I yelled at him to get out."

Again she pauses. "Of course, I didn't know he was dyin'.

"And we had good times together, too. Like when we built the house for Teddy on one of the shelves of his bookcase," she says, referring to Joey's old stuffed bear, the most loved and limp of his possessions. "And we cut the rug for the floor and glued the watch to the ceiling for a clock and all.

"Remember how he used to wire his room so if you guys opened the door his alarm clock went off? Well, I helped with that. I know I bossed him a lot, but when he was doin' things in his room, he bossed me, too."

If Peggie feels any guilt, it is because she does not grieve as Joe and I grieve. "I keep waitin' for it to hit me the way it has you guys, but it never does."

"We both got our ears pierced six months ago, right, Peg? Now look at your ears. You can hardly see where they were pierced. Then look at my gaping holes. Young people mend more quickly than older people. Be glad you're young."

I explain that a parent's sorrow for a lost child is uniquely heavy in the experience of human heaviness. That losing a brother is, in part, losing a rival. That she mustn't feel bad if now and then she even feels glad that all our attention, all our extra money is hers now.

Peggie scrutinizes my ear lobes. "How gross, mother. I mean, you can see the light clear through. And your ears are still gooey. Are your ears always going to be gooey?

"Now for goodness sakes, mother, I don't know what you're cryin' about this time, but if it's because you're still bound and determined that you weren't a good enough mother to Joey, instead of moanin' and groanin' about it, why don't you just do a better job on me?"

*　*　*　*　*

We take Peggie and her friend Gladys to see the Cleveland Indians play. Actually, for the girls a rock group performing after the game is the main attraction.

The improvement in Peggie's lungs when she was in the hospital was negligible. She's supposed to be sensitive to antibiotics she can take at home, but her improvement out of the hospital has been minimal as well. As time passes, Joe's and my panic over Peg becomes as chronic and convulsive as her cough.

"Are you getting tired?" we ask her as the game drags on. "Are you ready to go yet? Are you sure?"

Joey died because he got a virus. We must do everything in our power to keep Peggie from getting a virus. Adequate rest is a must.

As the game enters its thirteenth inning, we lead the girls from the stadium. "Let's listen to the game on the radio," Joe suggests brightly as we get in the car.

But Peg huddles in the far corner of the back seat and talks to Gladys in tones just loud enough for us to hear. "Boy, are my parents hyper about my health. Bein' up late one night isn't gonna kill me."

I know that most adolescents resent their parents worrying about them. They're not sure themselves that they can cope with their lives; their parents' worry compounds their own.

"How many deadly viruses do you think are stalking Cleveland in August?" I ask Joe, and we eye each other sheepishly.

"I'm sorry you were embarrassed in front of Glad over leaving the game and not hearing the rock group," I apologize to Peg as she gets ready for bed.

"I told Glad about Joey."

"Oh?"

"Yeah. I said, 'Did you know my brother died?' And she said, 'No.' And I said, 'Well, he did.' And she said, 'Oh.' I mean, I thought I should tell her. With me not seein' Gladie since school's been out, what if she didn't know? What if she said something about Joey and then I had to tell her? I waited till there was a lot of screaming and yelling. I told her during a home run."

All in all, it is harder for Peggie to handle Joe's and my reactions to Joey's death than her own. On Mondays, Joe's day off, he hovers over Peg. "Want to play three-handed solitaire?" he asks. And asks.

A little extra attention is fine, but too much attention is control. "You guys have gotta stop lookin' at me like I'm me and Joey both," Peg rages.

Last Monday we went to a "Love Bug" movie instead of playing solitaire. All at once Peggie's exuberant whisper carried above the hubbub on the screen. "Listen to mother. Did you hear her? She laughed! She really did. I heard her. Did you hear her, father? Mother laughed!"

* * * * *

Dr. Rathburn talks about putting Peggie in the hospital again, but she tells him she cannot miss the first week of ninth grade when everything is explained. She tells me she has never dreaded anything more than going back to school.

"I thought things got better last year, Peggie."

"Yeah, but better than what? You remember that concert I went to last year? Well, when I walked in the auditorium that night, I only saw one girl I knew, and that was Rose. Ya know, the one who always mocks me out. But I asked her if I could sit with her, and she said, 'Sure.'

"But then in a few minutes she said she forgot but she had to go to the choir room for something, and she might be back for intermission. And then she came right back and went and sat with these other kids.

"That was the loneliest I ever felt in my whole life."

Oh, Peggie. I'd not take that kind of risk myself.

"I did get invited to Denise's party though, mother. Now that was a good thing that happened. Remember how I was in that group that was talkin' about the party, and I said that the year before I invited Denise to my party, and they kept on talkin' about the party, and I said that the year before Denise invited me to her party, and the girl who was giving the party asked me did I want to come?"

Oh, Peggie. Why don't you take the easy way out and say you're too sick to go back to school?

"Well, that's the kind of thing I'm gonna do more of this year. There's nothin' about me people wouldn't like if they got to know me, is there? I'm goin' in there and I'm gonna make those kids like me. Right, mother?"

Wrong, Peggie. At least wrong on the first day of school.

"All the girls were giggling and askin' me if I bought my clothes at Winnie the Pooh," she moans, collapsing on the couch inside the front door. "And after Memphis grandmother spent $109.42 on my school clothes *upstairs* at the May Company! Ever since father read out of the Bible that time about our having heavenly bodies one day, I always thought of those clothes as my heavenly body clothes. Boy!

FOURTEEN YEARS OLD   29

"And not a single person noticed my new glasses." Joe and I had dipped into our Christmas fund to replace Peg's hated, outdated plastic frames with the coveted wires.

"And that Eugene. I guess he's given up on me dyin' right away, 'cause today he was telling everybody in homeroom that he read an article in *Reader's Digest*, and I was gonna die at twenty. And the kids in homeroom passed it all over band, and everybody was lookin' at me funny.

"Oh, mother, I prayed so hard that things would be nice, and they weren't nice, and I try and try to forgive Eugene, and I can't. You remember that group I was in in the sixth grade, and how Mary was in that group? Well, when she came in history today, I said, 'Want to sit with me, Mary?' and she said, 'No,' and went and sat on the other side of the room.

"Nobody wants to be around me when Eugene says the things he does.

"Ya know, there's one reason I think we should be really glad about Joey's dyin'. I mean, if he had to die, isn't it good he died before he had to go to junior high?"

For the past two years Joe has talked repeatedly to Eugene's counselors and homeroom teachers, who in turn have talked repeatedly to Eugene. Joe and I have both talked relentlessly to Peggie about how to handle her differentness and those like Eugene who capitalize on it. Everybody we know has talked to God about Eugene.

"The time to talk is over," decrees Joe, and he charges up the street like an avenging linebacker to a family in our church with a son at J.F.K. Junior High School—a large son. Joe explains the situation and suggests that the boy take care of Eugene in any way he sees fit.

"I can't believe he did that," shrieks an appalled, pleased Peg.

"I can't believe you did that, Joe. Is assault and battery the Christian way?"

"Lay off Peggie Woodson or I'll make you wish you had," our large ninth-grade friend growls at Eugene. It is as though he flips a switch and turns Eugene off. Eugene taunts Peggie once more and then never again.

"We should have done it two years ago," says Joe grimly. I weep with relief.

They are fighters, my husband and my daughter, open to special cruelty and singular conquest.

* * * * *

Peggie goes trick or treating one last Halloween. "I'm gonna do things up right, this bein' my last year and all," she announces, cutting away on her washing machine costume.

She sets off on the big night wearing one large box from her shoulders down and a smaller box on her head—the eye holes labeled *hot water–cold water;* the nose hole labeled *half full–full;* and the mouth hole, *delicate cycle.*

"Trick or treat," she cries, sticking her hand out of the door in the middle of the lower box. A front loader.

"I was a sensation," she gloats, dumping her loot on the floor inside the front door just as she and Joey had done together every year since they first tricked or treated as tiny children holding tightly to their daddy's hands. "Like this woman up the street takes one look at me standin' there and yells, 'Hey, Herman, come here. You gotta see this one.'"

How I admire that conscious or subconscious part of Peg that knows in every hard time what *must be done.*

And then her gerbils die. Jerbie and Gerbie have been old and suffering, but their deaths are catastrophic nonetheless. We have a burial for Jerbie, the first to go, on the creek bank in our back yard "in a wild, natural place he would have liked," Peggie's tears plip-plopping on the red and yellow leaves with which she covers the tiny mound.

Then she insists that Joe take Gerbie to the vet to be put to sleep, as the euphemism has it. Joe feels silly taking a gerbil to the vet to be put to sleep, but it is not the first silly thing he has done for the love of Peggie. The minute he leaves the house cradling the shoe box with those precious scramblings inside, Peg folds into uncivilized sobbing.

These gerbils were Joey's before they were Peggie's, the last living things we had of Joey's. Strange, though, how Peggie cries more hysterically for her gerbils than for her brother. Is it more tolerable to cry for a smaller loss than a friend-loss? Or is Peggie purging herself of all her griefs with this one Niagara of salt spray?

"Tomorrow," Peg dictates the minute Joe gets back to the house, "we will go out and buy new gerbils."

Peggie thinks she'd like to be a writer someday. "Not like you, mother," she's quick to add. "I mean, I'd like to look up everything on a subject and then organize it and write it out. I'd never want to be a writer like you, thinkin' stuff up out of my head and bein' rejected."

I haven't planned that Peg take after me in so many ways. I certainly haven't pushed her into loving words the way I do. I wish she didn't have to push me aside so energetically in order to become her own person. She knows I don't handle the rejection of my manuscripts well.

People repeatedly tell Peggie how much she and I look alike. "Oh, no!" she hollers. "Oh, no, no, no!

"Now don't go gettin' the wrong idea, mother," she soothes me, as though it is my habit to misinterpret her innocence. "It's not that I don't think you're good lookin'. I just don't wanna look like my mother, no matter what my mother looks like."

"Did you take your allergy pill today, Peg?" I ask.

"Yes, I took my allergy pill today. Did you take your mother pill today?"

"I don't need to take a pill to be a mother. Did you take your back-talk pill today?" Yet I think she has a point.

Recently she wrote a haiku for English.

> riders are guided
> by the day's "westering" light
> through exploding land

She picked some of the words out of a *National Geographic* she was reading at the time. Still, I am awed at how good the haiku is. I am also awed by the realization that the light of my motherhood should be a westering light these days. If only there were an anti-mothering pill on the market, to be taken in small doses as a child hits adolescence, and then in larger and larger amounts till the grown child's own sun hangs high in the sky.

* * * * *

W e've been home from Slippery Rock for a week now, a Thanksgiving convocation our denomination held a hundred miles from here in Pennsylvania. We took Denise along to keep Peggie company, busting our budget and getting the girls a room to themselves. "You're on your own, kids." "Free at last!" we hear the kids chanting through the wall that separates their room from ours.

They did attend Sunday worship with us. When the congregation gave the speaker a standing ovation, Peg leaned over to ask why everybody was standing up. I whispered back that this is the ultimate way an audience has of saying they appreciate who a person is and what he or she represents.

Today Peg wanders into my study and says, "You remember when we were at that conference and me and Denise went to that concert? Well, you and daddy wouldn't have liked it, because it was really hard rock, but they were classy musicians, mother.

"And they were playing and singing, and we were clapping, and they were playin' and singin', and we were clappin'. But then they stopped, and they said they appreciated our clapping for them, but that they really performed so people would clap for God, and that they were gonna be quiet for a minute and just let us do that—just let us clap for God.

"Well, I nudged Denise," Peg says, her eyes getting big with the bigness of what is to come. "And me and her, *we stood up*. Now we really stood out, mother, because everybody else was sitting down and there we were standing up, but I didn't care, 'cause for once in my life I knew I was doin' the right thing. That maybe never again would I do as right a thing, but that right then I was doin' it.

"And pretty soon everybody else was standing up, and we were all clappin' and clappin'. And we clapped so long and so hard, it felt like we were never gonna stop clappin' for God."

Then Peg looks at me, her face shining like the sun. "I bet God really liked that, don't you think so, mother? If I'd of been God, I'd have liked it. Oh, I just know He liked it."

Does she have to say good morning to everyone, or can she just silently shove the bulletins into people's hands? Is she supposed to start up the aisle to take the collection before the music starts, or is the music supposed to start before she starts up the aisle? I want to laugh at Peg's panic over such a simple thing as ushering in church on Youth Sunday, but I restrain myself.

"Becky thought for three weeks, and she couldn't think of anything to say for the offertory prayer. Finally daddy told her, and she wrote it on a card. If she looks like she's not used to wearing a dress, that's because they just bought her one last night." Neither Peggie's nor Becky's qualms are an act.

Becky comes home with us after church, and we hold a post-mortem. "We did the most female thing we could do," Peggie giggles. "We giggled. But I didn't drop the collection plate. Did anybody here see me drop the collection plate?"

The girls are so full of Youth Sunday, it is after dinner before Becky remembers her big surprise. Then she takes from her purse and with flourishes unwraps—ta-ta-ta-ta—John Denver's Coke can. "I borrowed it from this guy at school, who got it from his father, who was walking through the airport with John Denver when he got done drinking the Coke out of it. I have to give it back tomorrow."

I take a picture of the girls each holding John Denver's Coke can with one hand. "I know it's silly," laughs Becky. "Any perspiration or anything would be gone by now."

"I bet you think it's silly, don't you, mother?" asks Peg. "But I bet you wouldn't think it was so silly if it was—Eric Severeid's pencil!"

* * * * *

We open our presents early on Christmas morning, Peggie glorying in excelsis over receiving all the top items on her list: a clock radio, Probe, a French doll, religious jewelry, a Snoopy pencil sharpener, and a Betsey Clark diary.

Joe makes her Christmas when he doesn't discover his gift from her till all the other presents are opened. An umbrella, wrapped in white toilet paper and red ribbon and hanging on the mantel like a candy cane.

She gives me a cactus arrangement from The Swiss Colony. How long must she have saved for it? The message on the label reads: Peggie Smile Glow As You Grow.

New York grandmother and grandfather, with us for two weeks now, treat us to Christmas dinner at the Holiday Inn, and the desk clerk takes a snapshot of us all lined up in front of the big red sled in the lobby. Christmas is the day for family members who have been apart to come together again. All day I wait for Joey to run in and complete the Christmas picture.

Everyone else spends the afternoon playing dominoes and parcheesi. I try to enter in, but the tension in me only expands. Am I the only one who misses Joey? When Peggie will not cooperate for her evening therapy, I explode. "Joey never gave me this much trouble for therapy."

Peggie jumps down from the therapy table and sprints through the house. "Father, father! Did you hear what mother just said? She said Joey never gave her as much trouble as me. She compared me to Joey! She really did! Can you believe she did that?" She races back to me. "I can't believe you did that, mother."

Everyone in the house knows of my perfidy. Everyone for several houses around knows. Yet when Christmas is over and I am finally permitted to go to bed, I find a typed note on my pillow. Peggie's forgiveness, the best of my presents: *Thou art the mots wonderful mother in the whole world!!!!!*

Peggie's new Betsey Clark diary has a motto on the cover.

REMEMBERED JOYS ARE NEVER PAST.

Her first entry reads:

Dec. 25 "Remembered joys are never past." I shall prove this true in writing about Joey (among other things). I remember last year, we had presents for Teddy and friends. I made a yellow collor for Teddy and hat for Ms. Mildred, his wife. In Sears when we were buying a cube puzzle for Joey I had to hide it under my hat to get it over to the counter without Joey seeing it.

Last New Year's Eve me and Joey got up at midnight. We went in mother and father's room with pots and pans and spoons to bang on them and Daddy just kept saying "go away" over and over again. One year we went in and we had hot chocolate from a thermos. It had been made up ahead of time.

I was just playing with Teddy. He was dancing to the music like he used to do with Joey.

* * * * *

Grandmother and grandfather go home to Long Island the day after Christmas. Peg is bereft. Old Joey-wounds have opened during the holidays, and new sorrow oozes out.

I take her to the shopping mall to spend her Christmas money, and she seems to have a good time. We march from the mall through the parking lot with arms linked, chanting, *"I left—I left—I left my wife and my forty-eight kids. . . ."* I pray as I pace that no one I know will see me.

Yet how unlike herself Peggie is on the way home, bouncing and hollering in the back of the car. "Me and Joey always drew this imaginary line down the center of the back seat," she mourns. "He'd karate chop me if even my elbow went over the line."

I chant loudly, but I am not Joey.

We decide we need to do something big and different on Christmas vacation this year, and on the spur of the moment we take Aunt Lynn up on her offer to fly us to California.

We hang on cable cars and roam through Fisherman's Wharf in San Francisco. We drive across the desert to Las Vegas. "Oh, my, shut your eyes, Peg," Joe warns as we pass the billboards on the way into town.

"Sin city," exults Peg.

We only go to Las Vegas to see Hoover Dam and to catch a sightseeing plane for the Grand Canyon, but Peg and I talk Joe into letting us sightsee one casino for educational purposes. Joe chooses The Circus, which is billed as a family casino, but no sooner does he shepherd us in than he insists on shooing us out. He cannot find his way out, however, and we ogle our way up and down miles of gambling tables and slot machines.

Joe keeps thinking of how Joey would be reacting if he were with us. I forget for blissful moments that he is not. Peg assumes that he is at home and that she must bring him souvenirs. The specialness of the trip brings its special pain.

Yet I'm surprised at how much the trip diverts us from nothing-but-pain; at how much the newness and the interestingness of it, and the love that gifted us with it, heals.

Aunt Lynn takes us to movie and television sets and to the

Wax Museum and Knott's Berry Farm and to every elegant restaurant in Los Angeles. Peggie is weak and coughing nonstop, and Joe rents a wheelchair for her at Disneyland. "I've asked God to give us one year to get over Joey before anything happens to Peg," he confides to me as Donald Duck waddles by.

Peggie disdains the wheelchair all day but sits in it at night to watch the electric parade, her face flickering with wonder as a world of fantasy floats past. And then as the snails draw abreast, one of the giant green velour creatures breaks rank, snails over to her wheelchair, and bobs his feelers at her.

"It's all right, isn't it, father, that he dipped to me? He really did, ya know. That snail dipped to me. I mean, I know he did it because I was in a wheelchair, and I don't belong in a wheelchair, but I do have cystic fibrosis, and that's about equal to bein' in a wheelchair even if it doesn't show, so it's all right, isn't it?"

May God bless all lighted people who bow to young girls in wheelchairs.

*　*　*　*　*

All the nicest kids in the ninth grade are in advanced English, mother." It becomes a litany as the new year speeds by.

"Hi, Peg. How'd it go today?"

"Good, mother. Ya know, all the nicest kids in the ninth grade are in advanced English. I mean, Judy and John and Denise and Mary and Derrick and Glad and Maxi and Louis. And they all eat lunch together, and I eat with them. And good old-fashioned Judy walks to social studies with me, and Derrick talks to me in math."

"And how do you account for this great change in fortune?"

"It could be God. It could be threatening Eugene. And it could be these," she says, spreading her hands over her new jeans.

"And it could be all three, Peg. God works in all kinds of ways, even through blue jeans."

"Hey, yeah."

"They're an unusual bunch in advanced English," the counselor informs us. "They think of themselves as intellectuals and compete academically. Very odd at this age."

"I've never seen a group of kids with such high moral standards," Miss Saunders, the young English teacher, adds. "They're just plain straight kids. They cling to each other like drowning souls in a lifeboat."

"You do realize that I'm really in high school now, don't you, mother? That the grades I get in the ninth grade count for college and all? I'm sure gonna work hard in Miss Saunders's class. I mean, all the nicest kids in the ninth grade are in advanced English."

Peg weighs seventy-seven pounds when we go to the hospital for her two-month checkup, a gain of five pounds. Her cough is not improving, but neither is it getting worse. Hospitalization isn't mentioned.

"What happened?" I ask Dr. Rathburn.

"I don't know. Don't ask any questions. Don't change anything you're doing."

"Do you think me havin' friends has anything to do with it?" Peg presses.

I do think Peg's friends have something to do with it. I think her advanced English friends have pulled her into that lifeboat Miss Saunders talks about—that they are literally saving her life. I also believe they are an answer to many people's prayers for Peg. How I thank God that He answered, that His infinite heart was moved—moved to action by a schoolgirl's misery.

"Denise's sister who goes to Sub West says that last year when she was in the ninth grade, if you didn't get drunk or get high or swear or make out, you mostly sat by yourself. Did I tell you there's this one guy in the eighth grade we let hang out with us because he can't find anybody in the eighth grade like him? It sure is weird about advanced English, isn't it, mother?"

"It sure is, Peg. I mean, all the nicest kids in the ninth grade are in advanced English."

Peg spends a lot of time writing in her diary.

In Science me, Judy, one other kid, and Denise were in a group. We found Denise's locker combination. She tore it up. We pieced it back together. (Denise protesting) It was fun. Denise's locker number is 1917—point of information.

Today was a ½ day. School ended at 1:05. Judy came over. We found out that one of my stamps is worth $10.00.

There was a fight in the hall. Traffic was blocked for miles. Tammy was really tough. Me and John simply could not get through. I bought a horse poster and a mouse ring holder for Denise's party.

"I'm gonna be busy the next couple weeks," Peg tells me. "I'm gonna make each of my friends a Valentine present." She says *my friends* with such a proprietary air. "I'm gonna make each one a red stained-glass window that says *Let your love shine*. I'll have to make about twelve—ya know, for all *my friends*."

* * * * *

Peg and Joe and I take turns proofing the galleys of my first book, *If I Die at Thirty*,* a book of conversations Peg and I had when she was thirteen and first slammed up against her prospects for early death. When Peg finds an error, she puts a check above the word and draws a smile face at the beginning of the line.

While I was writing that book, I always told Peg that before the book went to press I would let her read it, and that I would delete anything she was unhappy with. Now, having read it, she doesn't say she likes the book, but she doesn't lift her voice in the expected lamentations either.

"Sometimes I have this daydream, mother. Like I have this Peggie Woodson column in the newspaper, and all the kids write in to tell me their problems. I mean, I know I talk off the top of my head, but I talk out of experience, too."

Any book about Peggie Woodson is beyond criticism.

"The only thing is, mother. Ya know all these deep-seated intellectual thoughts of mine you've written down that you like so much? Well, I don't think it's fair that people will know everything that's goin' on inside me when I won't know anything that's goin' on inside them.

"And another thing," she adds, her eyes hopping like two mischievous partners in a blue *Blue Danube Waltz*. "If it's my thoughts you've written down, who ought to get the money from the book? Me, right? Come on, mom, I know you're writing the book for God and people and all, but don't you think a little bit about havin' your name right in there and all that money?"

But at night as I stand beside her bed, Peg grabs my hand. "I don't really want to be famous and rich so much, mother. Just mostly to help people. I mean, I figure that's why I was born thinkin' different from most kids, so I could say the things I say in this book and help people understand it all—about why bad things happen and how not to be afraid of death. They shouldn't be all mixed up with different theories."

*Published in 1975 by Zondervan Publishing House. Published in paperback in 1977 under the title *It's Great to Have a God Who Cares*.

We are going to finish Joey's picture album today," Peg declares as we linger over Saturday noon hot dogs and apples. "You haven't put any pictures in it for three years, mother. And we're gonna keep remembering all the good times—not like some people act, like the dead person never existed. I mean, we gotta write down what Joey was like, 'cause I'm forgetting already."

"Remember that time we were playing four-handed solitaire and Joey won as usual?" asks Joe. "And he was preening himself as usual?"

"You mean that time you told him he better watch out 'cause pride goeth before a fall, and he kept on boastin', and he was squirmin' around so much that he fell off his chair? I never saw a proverb happen like that before."

"And remember that time he told us about at C.F. Camp when he went to Mass by mistake?" I join in. "Remember how they always took the Protestant kids into the woods for a service on Sunday morning, and the Catholic kids they loaded on a truck and took to Mass? And they kept asking Joey, 'What are you, Joey? What are you, Joey?' And he kept saying, 'Alls I knows I'm Christian,' and they put him in the truck."

"Boy, was he dumb. What are we anyway, father? I always get mixed up between Protestant and Presbyterian."

"Alls I knows we're Christian," chuckles Joe. "Maybe that Joey wasn't as dumb as you think, Peg."

"Now that's the kind of thing I mean about Joey," Peg gloats as we laugh together. "Wasn't that nice? Doesn't that make you feel better?"

Still, it is not a good day for me, and I am crying in the bedroom later when Peg walks in on me. She surveys the scene, sits down on the chair beside the bed, and promptly falls off it. I laugh so hard I have to stop crying. Every time I cry for the rest of the day, Peg crashes off whatever she's sitting on.

But I keep on crying. I make believe I have to do something in the basement, but Peggie follows me. "Ya know what I've decided, mother? That if you don't buy yourself a blazer with your money, I'm gonna buy you one with mine. You've wanted a blazer for so long. I want you to have one, mama.

"You don't believe me when I say my comments about your not being a good mother, do you? Don't you say comments sometimes that you don't mean?"

I continue to cry, but more now for Peggie than for Joey, for what I am doing to her and for what she is trying so hard to do for me. How will I ever survive without the common sense she tells me and the sweet comfort she distills—when it is for her I grieve?

I keep feeling that what Peggie does is not right because it agrees with what all the grief books say, but that the grief books are right because they agree with what Peggie does.

How ungrown and unguarded—and how graced—she looks tumbling off chairs in her Charlie Brown nightshirt. With her skinny arms and her innate wisdom wrapped around me, Peggie is pulling me through.

*   *   *   *   *

Will you promise me something?" Peg demands, plopping on the bed where I lie reading.

"What?" I counter warily.

"Will you promise you'll give me a week's notice when I'm dying?"

I think I've adjusted to Peg's at-ease attitude toward death, but I have to hold my heart at stiffest attention to keep it from total collapse. "Would you want to tell me why a week's notice is important to you, honey?"

"Well, ya know how Judy has always admired my *Basically I'm a warm person* button? I'd like to have time to give it to her, and I'd like to make Betsey Clark pictures for my other friends. It'd be kind of like graduating from junior high, signin' yearbooks and all. I'd like to finish it up right.

"Then, too," she adds, "you know how I'm always readin' *Campus Life* magazine and how it helps me be a Christian and all? Well . . . if I die in junior or senior high, I'd like to send a subscription of *Campus Life* to . . . uh . . . Eugene."

I gape. Eugene, her arch-tormentor?

"Well, mother," Peg huffs. "Somebody has to do something about creeps like Eugene."

There. She has made out her will, so to speak, and forgiven her enemy. Are her preparations for death now complete?

She begins to cough, and I sit up and shelter her in my arms. How does such a blow-away body endure the force of such spasms? The touch of my hands is light, but the clutch of my heart is mother-fierce.

When I think of this year in which Peggie was fourteen, I think of it as the year in which Joey died. I will never think of it in any other way.

But Peggie already refers to it as "the year of ninth grade English," the year of the good rather than the bad. The year she determined she would survive Joey's death and by God's grace did. The year she determined she would not die and by God's grace lived—with friends.

What a fearsome will resides in such a frail frame. When God made Peggie Woodson in His image, did He specialize in her that sacred stubbornness of His that keeps Him from ever giving up on us?

Whenever Peg remembers the purchase of her first bra, she remembers only the laughter that bounced from cubicle to cubicle.

Fifteen Years Old

For her birthday, Joe gives Peggie a Good News Bible with a denim cover, and I give her a Snoopy-Woodstock banner. Snoopy and Woodstock sit at the bottom of the banner looking at each other and going "Hee Hee Hee Hee Hee." Peg folds it up among her books and takes it to school.

I drove for an hour to get the banner at a store over beyond the hospital where Peg spied it after a recent doctor's visit. I hate that stop-and-go trip, but I would travel further than that to get Peggie the thing she wants most in the world for her birthday.

I worry during the day that Peggie isn't aware of the love that inspires so much that Joe and I do for her. Most of us parents would lay down our lives for our children, but do we ever tell them? I tell Peg when she comes home from school.

"Oh, for goodness sakes," she scorns, "don't go makin' a big thing out of it."

But I'm glad I told her anyway.

"You know what happened at lunch today, mother? Well, Judy brought this doughnut and stuck a candle in it, and everybody sang to me. I mean, she really baked me a special low-fat cake, but she dropped it before she got it out of her apartment, so she brought the doughnut instead. And all my friends gave me presents. I never got so many presents."

Then before Peg can finish displaying her bounty, the doorbell rings, and there on our little porch stand Miss Murdock, her sixth grade teacher, and Aunt Kate from church, and Mary from up the street—all bearing gifts.

"How about that?" exults Peg. "A traffic jam in the driveway on my birthday." And her manner adds, *Now that is a big thing, mother.*

I'm as happy for Peg for this first birthday on which friends reach out to her as Peg is happy for herself, but I'm surprised at how shut out I feel, too. As long as Peggie didn't have friends, she had to have me. Now even my banner is important to her only because "all the kids were looking at it and going *hee hee hee.*"

Joe is taking us to the Pancake House for supper, and Glad, Peg's old friend from school, is to go with us. But before we leave to pick her up, Peg gets her first menstrual period. "On my birthday," she wails. No amount of talk about God's wonderful plan for women pacifies her. "If God's creation is so wonderful, why doesn't He fix it so you don't have to start with this mess till you're ready to have a baby?"

"You mean so you could push a button when the time is right?"

Peggie giggles. "Well, something like that."

She pulls me into her bedroom and takes Teddy down from his shelf. "Are you at the point where you can say *Hi* to Teddy yet, mother?"

"Hi, Ted."

"Hi, grandma."

Peg bundles into her light blue parka, its white fur framing her flushed birthday-girl face. The parka's bulk camouflages her body's wraithlikeness, but other aspects of her littleness Peg is not ready to leave behind. "Ya know," she says as she skates down the drive on the ice, "it's harder and harder for me to think of Teddy as a live animal and easier and easier for me to think of him as stuffed. Isn't that terrible?"

"No, Peg. That's fifteen."

* * * * *

Joe goes out of town for the weekend, and Peg and I go out on the town, to the Sveden House smorgasbord —twice. On each visit Peg makes her way down the buffet with a ransacking appetite—thrice. "I'm always tellin' ya there are advantages to me having C.F.," she laughs.

"Will that be separate checks?" the waitress asks on our second excursion. What a good mood that puts Peggie in.

I ask Peg why she thinks we don't have long, serious conversations any more the way we did when I was writing *If I Die at Thirty*.

"Because I don't have any problems any more, ya know? I mean, what would we talk about? If you want us to have conversations again, we're gonna have to discuss your problems."

"You think I have more problems than you do?"

"Tell me about your problems."

"Well, sometimes I feel alone, even when I'm with a lot of people. I think differently than most people I know, and I read different books. I don't like being lonely, but it seems I have to be willing to be what I am if I'm going to make my unique contribution."

"Now just listen to you, mother. Of course you're gonna be lonely. How many people do you know who walk around talking about making their unique contributions? Now what you have to do is make an effort, make an effort, mother, to find other people like you. I mean, have you thought about taking an English course at Baldwin Wallace College, something that would correspond to advanced English for me?"

I tell Peg that I keep thinking I should write another book about her, that I go on scribbling down the good stuff she says out of habit, and that it seems a shame to let it go to waste.

"Well, if you do write another book, I hope you'll make me sound older in this one, ya know? You always make me sound like such a little kid."

"I've been listening carefully to you today, Peg. You still say *I mean* a lot. I listened for that because I used that as an identifying tab in *If I Die*. But you say *ya know* a lot, too."

"Yeah, a lot of kids do. Last year this kid in history said it so often I sat there and counted. I wish I didn't say it so much."

"Well, if you ever want my help, I'll remind you when you do. Just say the word."

"Oh, would you, mother?"

I tell Peggie that I'll help her not to say *ya know* so often if she can think of something she can do to help me stay on my diet.

"I could tickle ya," suggests Peg gleefully, and the deal is set. "And you have to come to me for permission if you want to go off your diet, right? I can't believe it! Do you know how important that makes me feel? Oh, boy! Tickle, tickle, tickle!"

* * * * *

Peggie has an extra good checkup. Partly because she talks Dr. Rathburn into doing his yo-yo tricks for her—and nobody can do yo-yo tricks like Dr. Rathburn—and partly because she has gained another three pounds.

She grand-dames through the waiting room. Eighty! She weighs eighty pounds! How long she has worked toward this magic number. "I don't want to buy too many new clothes right away, though," she tells me in a sober aside. "I mean, what if I get thin again?"

But then her somberness gives way to temper. "I shouldn't have even told you, mother. You know how you are. Now you'll go getting all upset if I don't always weigh that much."

Peg's goal for the school year has been to miss no days of school except for trips to the doctor, and so far she has met that goal. "Mary misses a lot more days than me," she brags. "Most kids miss more days than me. It's amazing how many kids have elbows that go out. Isn't it good that I haven't missed·any days, mother?"

The car has been bucking and stalling of late, and we say a little prayer as we leave the hospital that we will not get stuck so far from home. At the first red light the car bucks and stalls. As I press the gas, I rock back and forth in that silly way drivers have of trying to make a car move. Peg rocks back and forth beside me, and under her breath I hear her imploring, "Go, God. Go, God."

The car goes. I look down at all eighty pounds of Peggie stomping the floor and cheering beside me, and I think, Go, God. Don't let Peg start missing days of school again and losing weight again. Please, God, keep on going.

*   *   *   *   *

Can you show me a verse in the Bible that will explain to Denise why I don't go to movies with a lot of not-nice stuff in them?"

"Well, let's see. How about this verse in Philippians?

Finally, brethren, whatever is true, whatever is honorable, whatever is just, whatever is pure, whatever is lovely, whatever is gracious, if there is any excellence, if there is anything worthy of praise, think about these things."

"Are you makin' that up? Does it really say that?" Peg grabs a paper napkin and scribbles *Philippians 4:8* in one corner.

Then she takes a piece of her daisy stationery, sits down at my typewriter, and slowly pecks out the verse, centering it vertically and horizontally. She makes one copy for me, one for Denise, and one to keep in the front of her school loose-leaf binder. She decoupages the verse and hangs it over her bed next to a blown-up photo of John Denver.

Actually, her room is papered with bookmarks that muse about birds that sing, not because they have answers but because they have songs, and posters that flourish friendship and faith and all things bright and beautiful. "It's all so uplifting, mother," she croons.

"Ya know why I like *Campus Life* magazine so much? Well, because it has the best cartoons for one thing, and because it's so well-written it makes me jealous. And it has articles to read if you want to think and articles to read if you don't. I mean, I get uplifted by almost every one, and it has this column on sex that doesn't make me feel like sex is dirty."

Friends take Peg and me to visit an apple farm on the outskirts of town. The farm sells hot apple cider and hard country candy and all kinds of Early American items. I expect Peg to be enraptured with it all, but she spends the whole time in the greeting card department copying down the verses. Like,

A house is a home
When love is there;
A soul is a temple
When filled with prayer.

At one point she motions wildly to me to join her. "Look, mother. This one is for you."

> The will of God
> will never lead you
> where the grace of God cannot keep you.

The thought that one day she may put Joe and me through what she has seen us go through over Joey is the primary thing about her own death that continues to bother her.

I am looking for some Betsey Clark wrapping paper for Peg when a representative of the Betsey Clark Company asks me what appeal the little old-fashioned girl with the long dresses and quaint sayings has for me.

I tell him that it is my daughter who is taken with his products, that they are one way she has of lifting herself above the four-letter words and obscene gestures of her generation.

The interviewer's pencil hesitates over his form.

"Just say it's innocence calling through the centuries to innocence," I tell the hapless young man.

"You know how the kids in school used to say *groovy* or *cool* or *neat* to describe something nice?" Peg asks. "And then they said *decent* or *tough*? Well, I been noticing they don't have a word like that any more. I think it's because for a lot of kids there's nothing nice left that you need a word like that for—like everything's polluted.

"You know what some girls in science were doing the other day, mother? They were calling from across the room, 'Are you a virgin, Peggie? Hey, Peggie, are you a virgin?' And I didn't answer, and they were laughin' and yellin', 'Hey, Peggie prostitute!'"

Suddenly Peg's face has a moist, tender look that reminds me of the grass that grows under the big shade tree in our back yard, a gentle-green grass, mossy and vulnerable. "What is a virgin anyway, mother? . . . Oh? Well, that's what I thought."

Then just as suddenly the grass is strong and thick and Crayola-green again. "Ya know, mother, there's one thing I'm really glad about it all, and that's that I don't have to worry about ever being raped. I mean, if anybody ever tried to rape me, I'd just yell, 'Not me, not me. I don't know how to do it!'"

*   *   *   *   *

A couple weeks ago in English we were discussing whether there were any honorable people left in the world, and I didn't say anything, but I was thinking, *There must be, 'cause I know two of them."*

We are sitting around the supper table, and I can see by the look on Joe's face that he, too, is going into shock. We are so used to put-downs these days that such high praise seems an unnatural act.

"I mean, sometimes I wonder where I'd be without you guys. I wouldn't have nothin' to look forward to but rotting in the ground. I was thinking about that today, it being Easter and all."

But when Joe holds family discussion a trifle too long after supper, Peg reverts to form. "Do you guys realize that in three years I'll be eighteen—old enough to move out of here?"

Later in the evening she sits on my lap examining the Easter book I gave her. *To Peggie from mother* I wrote on the flyleaf. "Whaddya mean *mother?"* Peg spouts. She crosses out *mother* and makes me write in *mama*. She hardly ever calls me *mama* any more. "Did you look a long time for the little book? Who says you can't buy love?"

Actually, the little book was put together backward, and I got it for seventy-five cents.

But we are anathema again when Peg scrambles down from my lap and finds herself outvoted when it comes to watching "The Six Million Dollar Man." "Ya know, it's funny, but every week when I'm in school all day, I forget how bad it is around here on weekends. Boy, it sure will be good to be back with normal people tomorrow."

Joe says I had best stop complaining about Peg's ambivalence. That I don't really want her to make up her mind about whether she's staying or walking away, because once she decides, there's not a doubt in the world about where her knee-socked, resolute legs will take her.

* * * * *

Peggie makes her first trip to the dermatologist. Strange things are happening to her face.

"It's acne on her forehead," says the doctor. "On her cheeks it's a reaction to the acne medicine she's been using, and on her nose it's exzema."

"But I don't put acne medicine on my cheeks," Peg objects.

The doctor explains that substances put on one area of the skin travel to other areas of the skin. He prescribes several ointments, and a nurse pops all Peg's pimples.

We stop in the ladies' room when it is over. Peggie's face, looking back at her from the mirror, is covered with blood and bewilderment. How will she ever show that face at school? If she asks, I will let her stay home for a few days.

She slumps into the car beside me, a damp lump of crumpled humanity. "I'm gonna ask father to buy me a ring with a cross dangling from it," she tells me in tired tones, "so I can remember I'm a Christian in the ninth grade."

* * * * *

The creeps were all seeing how much noise they could make during the lectures, squeaking their shoes on the new floors and all. Me and Judy were the only ones interested in the paintings." So Peg reports on her French class's trip to the art museum.

I suggest to Peg that maybe she has an unusual interest in art.

"I have an interest in anything I don't know, mother. I just want to learn anything there is to learn, even math, and you know how I hate math. But math is the one course that you're always learnin' altogether new stuff in.

"So what if everybody else can do a problem in ten minutes and it takes me an hour? So what if I'm never gonna use it? Oh, mother, I hope the time never comes in all my life when I'm not going to school, at least not taking a course someplace.

"Did you know there's no such thing as a line? The teacher told us about it in art the other day. I mean, you draw two planes coming together with different shades of light and dark, but you never draw a line. Isn't that the most fascinating thing? I just get so excited when I learn something new. It doesn't happen too often, though. It's like school tries to take that out of you."

"Miss Saunders says she can't believe the contributions you make in advanced English, Peg."

"Yeah, but that's just with Miss Saunders and with those kids. In other classes I work at not sayin' anything smart, because it sets you apart, and the kids would all laugh. A lot of them could say smarter things than me, but they think it's dumb to be smart."

Peg gets so worked up over the whole learning bit that when her father comes home later that night, she drags him to the kitchen window. "You must know," she stammers, shaking Joe, her red Mother Hubbard nightgown swirling about her slight form in playful frenzy. "The stars, I mean. All those constellations you can't even imagine. They must be there for some purpose. If you're a minister and you don't know, who would know? What's out there do you think?"

Peggie fastens a picture of Jesus to the refrigerator door with her *Happiness is contagious. Be a carrier.* magnet. He's throwing His head back and laughing for all He's worth.

"That's my favorite picture of Jesus," she maintains. "All the other pictures of Him are so dumb. I mean, He looks so timid, like He's afraid to enjoy life. Wouldn't you be embarrassed if somebody from India came over here and you had to show him one of those pictures and say 'That's my God'?

"But here the way He's laughing I bet He sounds just like father sounds in the movies when he laughs so hard everybody starts laughin' at father laughin'.

"You know why I'm so crazy about that yellow blouse I bought to go with my black pants? Because it's so bright. Don't you just love bright, cheery things? You know how I'm gonna decorate my apartment when I'm eighteen and I move out of here? All yellow and white. Can you imagine how sunshiny that will be?"

Smile faces have decorated our mantel for as long as I can remember, but increasingly Peggie's own face is smiling. She has always read avidly, but this mania for learning she's exhibiting lately is a step beyond. There's a kind of impurity she never knew existed before, so how could she have pitted herself against it as she's doing now?

I have the feeling that this year in which Peggie is fifteen will be a year of enlargement for her. Joey's death and her own crisis fight to live have waylaid her in her growing up, but now that these things are behind her to some extent, it's as though Peggie Woodson cannot wait to affirm the substance of Peggie Woodson.

"I still want to be a research writer, mother. You know how I like to look stuff up and organize it. But I want to be the kind of research writer that, when she puts it all together, makes something new out of it, something that will be a part of me that I can give away to other people."

Judy's mother tells me she overheard Peg and Judy talking about careers. "I may have problems when I get in my twenties," Peggie said, "because I'll probably be in the hospital a lot. But, then, who knows? I may be too busy to be in the hospital."

She watches a favorite actress being interviewed on television, a real star.

"What is the most basic thing you hope to accomplish in life?" asks the host.

"To become a superstar," says the star.

"That's it?" snorts Peg. "A superstar? That's all she wants to be? I just lost my respect for her, mother."

* * * * *

Peg's squealing on the phone last night rose to pig pitch. I thought something sensational must be happening to Peg, but it was John telling her that a senior girl had asked him to the prom. John, from ninth grade advanced English, is Peg's best friend-who-is-a-boy.

Then this morning Peg wakes up with the pain she gets in her stomach whenever she's distraught. It seems that yesterday at school a girl confided to Peg that her parents hate her boyfriend; that every time she goes out with him, her mother says she can tell from her father's breath that his ulcer is getting worse; that his ulcer will surely rupture during her next date. So the girl can't see the boy any more, and she is crazy about him.

"Why am I like this, mother?" Peg groans, clutching her own ulcer area. "Once on 'Star Trek' they had a woman called an empath. Is that what I am?"

We can't find *empath* in the dictionary. We look up *pity* and *sympathy* and *compassion*, but Peg wants a word that means feeling with people when they're happy as well as sad.

We try our thesaurus and come up with *fellow-feeler*. "That's you, Peggie. That's it."

"It makes me sound like a bug," she giggles. "Or a pervert. But why am I like this? Is something wrong with me?"

I tell Peg that nothing is more right than one human spirit uniting itself with another, but I warn her that pain is inherent in that kind of loving.

"Yeah, but it's a lot more fun, too."

Once Peggie willed to find a friend; now she wills to be one.

* * * * *

What do you think the primary influence on your Christian growth has been, Peg?"

"Well, for one thing I think it's been having somebody to answer my questions. I mean, I'm really spoiled. You want to know anything out of the Bible, you just ask father. He tells you—poof, poof!"

Bless Joe, I think, who so often sets aside the questions he thinks Peggie ought to be asking at family discussion and instead conducts a theological analysis of something like "why all the kids have so much fun making fun of the boy who's wimpy."

"And I'll tell you another thing," Peg adds. "Most kids these days swear a lot, but I don't swear, right? Well, what would happen if I walked into this house and said a nice fat swear word? Can you imagine the look on father's face? I mean, what chance do I have to be a swearer when the worst thing anybody around here says is *doggone it?*

"And you know how father's always prayin' all the time? Ya know, I was thinkin' the other day that father doesn't do that to teach me to pray on every occasion. He does that because that's the way he is. Like he's always jumpin' up and turnin' off the TV if the women aren't wearing enough clothes. You married a weird person, mother.

"And I'm not allowed to watch game shows because they might instill greed in me. Now I might not like that, but I understand it. Sometimes I try to explain it to the kids at school."

Peg is quiet for a minute. "Daddy's 100 percent for God, isn't he?"

Then she thinks again. "Whadaya mean, what did you guys do to help me be a Christian? Who says you guys did anything? Being a Christian comes naturally to me."

"I hope I never let her down," says Joe.

* * * * *

I know I am too old to have another child, but I see a gynecologist and ask his opinion anyway.

"I've delivered healthy babies from older women than you," the doctor says. "I don't advise it, but if you are set on it, get pregnant. Then at three months have a genetic consultation. If it looks as though the fetus may be defective, abort."

I rage at people everywhere who would, if they had had their way, have flushed my Joey and my Peggie down the drain. Don't they realize that children with no legs climb to alpine heights more often than children who are whole? They may be sick in body, but the whole world's soul is sounder because of them.

During her last hospitalization, Peg made a friend of a beautiful, dark-haired, miniature girl with C.F. named Bonnie. Bonnie gave Peggie a poem she had written on one of the hospital's paper napkins. Bonnie is eleven and weighs thirty-five pounds.

> I have cystic fibrosis
> It is a lung disease
> This hurts your lungs really bad
> It makes you cough and wheeze
>
> It makes my mucus really thick
> It clogs up my air sacs
> It's everywhere down in my lungs
> And these are the simple facts
>
> The thing that is really bad
> I catch the things you don't
> Like bacteria, staph, and other bugs
> That can't come out or won't
>
> Every day I take lots of pills
> To fight those awful germs dead
> To help those pills a little bit
> I say my prayers before bed
>
> And I take lots of mist every day
> To make my mucus thinner
> And if I get to coughing a lot
> I might barf up my dinner

The older we get, the worse our lungs
So we may die a little young
But Spirit we have
And Spirit we got
And I can darn well tell ya
We have a heck of a lot!!!

"She reminds me of me when I was her age," says Peg. "Precocious. Have you noticed that the older I get the less smart things I say?

"You know what Bonnie told me? She told me that when she was little, she was sick all the time, and she hurt so badly she cried all the time. And the only time she stopped crying was when her mother rocked her and sang to her, and only then when she sang her songs of Jesus. I bet you could write a book about a lot of kids with C.F., mother."

The school year, in fact Peggie's whole sojourn in junior high, is drawing to a close. "I've got some stuff here for the memory box," she tells me. "Here, let me show you." She goes over each item.

A letter from her principal congratulating her for her clarinet performance in the Cleveland Instrumental Solo and Ensemble Contest. Progress reports from various teachers who have written in one way or another that Peggie is a fine student and a pleasure to have in class. A ribbon awarded her for outstanding service as a movie ticket taker. Programs from two band concerts. A *Go, Panthers! Sock it to 'em* banner. And a letter from the principal congratulating her on being one of five students whose names will be inscribed on a permanent plaque in the hall for having achieved an A average for three years at J.F.K. Junior High.

* * * * *

I tell Peg that the main thing that has gotten me to the end of this endless year has been having a purpose in life large enough to hold even an event as immeasurable as Joey's death—wanting Joey's death, if he had to die, to glorify God.

Joey died one year ago today.

"Where in the Bible does it say anything about the purpose of our lives being to glorify God?" Peg's words jump at me, angry for response.

My mind isn't working well right now, and I cannot think of where. "We'll ask daddy, Peg."

I do tell her about the first question in the old Westminster Catechism: *What is the chief end of man? The chief end of man is to glorify God and enjoy Him forever.* And about a little, very friendly boy in our last church who was studying the child's version of the catechism and approached strangers on the street corner asking: "Who made you? What else did God make? Why did God make you and all things?"

"Why God made you is the most important question you can ever ask, Peg."

We try to come up with a way of expressing the concept of giving glory to God in everyday words, language that will get it down to where people's longings are, but in the end we decide that if there is not a better question to ask, maybe there is not a better way to answer it either.

"Unless it might be 'clapping for God,' Peg."

Peg looks at me awe-struck. "Like at the rock concert, mother? Boy, I do all kinds of good stuff without knowin' it. How about that? I did my purpose without even knowing I was doin' it."

I recall for Peg a passage in a book I read recently, *One Day in the Life of Ivan Denisovich* by Alexandr Solzhenitsyn, the story of one day in the life of a man in a Russian labor camp. Toward the end of the book the hero turns to the man in the cot next to him, a Baptist, and says, "It works out all right for you, Alyosha. You are sitting here in this prison for Jesus Christ's sake. But for whose sake am I here?"

"I sit beside Joey's grave, Peg, and I think of his body down there in his blue cowboy pajamas with the left foot sewed back together, covered with his red and blue quilt, and I wonder whatever I would do if I had no one for whose sake I could sit there."

"Well, I hope daddy can find a couple of verses that put it all plain. How could you not know something like that, mother?" Peg turns an accusing back to me and runs from the room.

But I know Peggie. The tears she is trying to hide do not stem from my insufficiency. She has a way of recognizing the primordial at first glance, my Peggie, and of racing after it, the tears on her cheeks glistening with illumined innocence.

* * * * *

Joe brings Peg and Becky back from church camp, Becky being Peg's best church friend. Church camp was pivotal to Joe's and my Christian growth when we were young, and we want Peg to have the same kind of experience we did.

She doesn't.

"The girls weren't interested in anything but boys, mother. I mean, all they did all week was flirt and go around with green eyelids and their belly buttons showing." Peg stands in the drive surrounded by duffel bag and bedroll, waving her sun-scorched arms in outrage.

"They made you go swimming, mother. One day there was actually this dead fish on the shore, and they made me go in the water. And they were always playin' volleyball, and I wasn't good at anything."

"We should have anticipated it," I tell Joe. "We tried to communicate Christianity to Peggie through a medium that was right for us, and for most girls her age, instead of a medium in which she feels at home." I think about the kind of kid Peg is. What does she enjoy? What reaches her mind and heart? Well, books, of course.

I've just finished reading *Eighteen—No Time to Waste*, an account of the death of one young girl and how her death brought many of the kids in her high school, the kind of kids Peggie calls creeps, to Christian faith. I leave the book on the coffee table in the family room.

Peg spends all night with her nose in the book as though she cannot breathe deeply enough of her native air. "You remember how toward the end of school I told you about my locker bein' stuck?" she asks when she puts the book down at last. "And how Eugene came along and said he'd open it and what was my combination? And I wouldn't tell him?

"I mean, I sure wasn't gonna give him the combination to my locker. And he fiddled around with it anyway and finally got it open. Well, I been thinking—it's too bad we couldn't add that story to *If I Die At Thirty*. I mean, the one nice thing he ever did for me."

Friends lend us their trailer for a few days of our vacation. Peggie doesn't want to come with us to the trailer; Peggie just wants our whole vacation to be over so she can get back to her friends. We remember that we didn't want to go places with our parents when we were fifteen, but it hurts anyway, this first time Joe and I go on vacation alone.

We leave Peg at home with Becky, who is two years older, and thirty dollars, and Becky's mother, who agrees to look in on them.

"I'm havin' the time of my life!" Peg screams into the phone when we call from our wilderness sojourn. "I finished Personal Typing. My highest score was 32/2. Of course Mary got 45. If she doesn't stop talkin' about it, I'm gonna send her back to California. Me and Becky are goin' to the Sveden House tonight. We haven't had one fight."

The pleasure Peg gets from sharing her good time away from us with us takes some of the stiffness out of me. What relaxes me even more, though, is her concern for our having a good time.

"Is daddy tense? You're sure? He's not worried about anything?" Usually she reacts with belligerence to her father's preoccupations. "Are you being bitten with mosquitoes, mother? Did you divide up the chores? Good, I knew you would."

When it is time for us to come home, Peg and Becky decorate the house, hanging crepe paper and WELCOME HOME signs from every hanging spot.

* * * * *

Ya know, mother, even if I miss you a little when I move out of here, I'll tell you one thing I won't miss, and that's your nagging."

Shock and self-defense! I am not a nagger!

I remember a conversation we had on Peg's thirteenth birthday.

"I don't think you really turned into a teenager today, Peg. I think you turned into a teenager a year or two ago."

"I think you're right, mother, 'cause you sure turned into the nagging mother of a teenager a year or two ago."

What is it about adolescents that turns perfectly winsome mothers into witches? The fact that they are withdrawing from our sphere of influence, and we're afraid they won't pay attention to us unless we keep after them? Are we getting back at them for their rejection of us? Are we disappointed in them in this in-between period of awkwardness?

"I would think you would have caught on by now," Peg scorns, "that when you say something to me in your remind tone, I automatically tune you out."

Whatever the cause of our nagging, it doesn't result in much.

Still, I don't think I do nag Peggie. Don't I let her live in a room without form and void with darkness on the face of the deep if that is what she chooses to do? And it is. I have never worked so hard at anything as at building up Peg's concept of herself.

But Peg sees things differently. "You make me feel like I never do anything around here, never do one single thing to help. And I do. You know how you say I'm always putting you down? Well, you should listen to yourself. You're always putting me down, always getting in your digs."

I decide to do as Peggie asks, and for three weeks I listen to everything I say to her and to everything my listening keeps me from saying to her. True, I don't hound her to clean her room, but I lose track of the number of times I comment on how glad I am her room is upstairs at the end of the hall. I am appalled by the impatience and comparison and ridicule I use as weapons on Peg.

"I don't know, Peg. You want to be treated like an adult, but you surely don't act like an adult."

"Peggie, will you please set this table?" Tone implying that if I don't pester her, the table will never get set.

"Boy, Peggie. You say you won't marry anybody who doesn't share the housework with you, but I don't see you sharing it with me."

"Becky's mother says that when she told Becky she was having discussion group at her place, Becky cleaned the whole apartment without being asked."

"You call this picked-up?"

May my moments of truth never stop nagging me.

* * * * *

Our church sponsors two Vietnamese refugees, Xuong and Thi. Actually, it's Aunt Kate and Uncle Jim who take them into their home. Joe and Peggie and I go with our friends to the halfway house to interview the young men.

"Where you live?" Xuong asks as we sit down together.

"Parma," Uncle Jim replies. "Near Cleveland."

Xuong turns to Thi. "You want to go?"

"But isn't there anything else you want to know first?"

"When we go?"

Later we learn that no one slept at the halfway house that night as all through the wee hours Xuong and Thi paraded through the halls chanting their joy. And the next morning when Uncle Jim was late coming for them, they funeral-marched through the same halls wailing, "Sponsors not come. Sponsors not come."

Peg watches the proceedings with her warm heart heated to the burning point.

She cries when she hears of Xuong's and Thi's reactions as they walk into their new home for the first time. "We very happy. Ah, this big place. You very kind. We call you mom and dad?"

And she laughs when she hears how they unpack, placing all their possessions on the closet shelf. Then, realizing that the dresser must be there for some purpose, positioning a bar of soap in the top drawer, a pencil in the middle drawer, and a handkerchief in the bottom drawer.

"I felt uneasy at first," Peg acknowledges as she comes home from her first evening with the Vietnamese. "But not for long. You know what Xuong calls me instead of Peggie? Pepsi! I mean, they don't even look Oriental."

"Oh? So small, with that straight black hair and slanted—"

"Well, mother, they may have looked Oriental when I got there, but they sure didn't look Oriental when I left."

How glad I am that our church provides people who bring this kind of experience into Peggie's life.

Then Mr. Nash, one of the older members of our church family, dies. It was Mrs. Nash we were expecting to die, strapped in a wheelchair as she's been for years now in a mental institution—an ancient shrew without substance or sound save for her rumpled skin and bent bones and loud curses.

For years Mr. Nash has been saying, "She's still the most beautiful woman in the world to me." A friend who lives in the apartment underneath him says she hears him crying all night, every night, in the vacantness above her.

"Now that's the kind of love you should get married for," says Peg.

His doctor tells Mr. Nash it's too much for him to make the trip to the institution, to fight the traffic and the heat, that Mrs. Nash doesn't know when he's there. But he makes the trip one more time and falls dead in the lobby of the hospital.

Joe has his funeral. "Make sure you tell our people that that was a good way for him to die," says Peg.

* * * * *

Peg sits on my lap in the big black chair. "You know, high school is different," she observes. "The cree—oops, I mean, the toughies stay by themselves. They leave the other kids alone. Like everybody knows where they belong. Did you hear that, mom? Toughies. Pretty good, huh?"

I have suggested many times that Peg find a word to describe the kids to whom she cannot relate that is descriptive without being judgmental.

"Mmm. Toughies, eh?"

"Promise you won't laugh if I tell you something, mother?"

"Promise." No way am I going to miss the good stuff that follows such a question.

"Well, you know how about a week before high school started, I was getting awful nervous about finding my way around the building, and the computer marked my program *irreconcilable conflict* and all, and I started getting those stomach aches again? Well, one night I couldn't sleep with a stomach ache, and I told God if He was ever gonna heal me, now would be a good time, and I haven't had a stomach ache since. And that's really weird, upset as I've been."

"Ve-dy in-de-res-ding, Peg."

"I mean, I was awful the way I asked Him. '*If* you're *ever* gonna do it, you might just do it now.' And nothing happened right away, and I forgot about it."

"Ve-dy, ve-dy in-de-res-ding, Peg."

Peggie grins. "What's gotten into you, mother?"

I hate to break up such a companionable time, but it is a school night and way past time for Peg to be in bed. A second before I call the hour to Peg's attention, she makes a move to get up. "I'll go, mother," she says haughtily. "But only if you admit that I moved before you spoke. Oh, wait. I got a better idea. Tell me to stay."

"You stay right here, Peggie Woodson. Don't you dare go to bed."

"I'm going to bed whether you like it or not." Peg can't help laughing at herself as she gets up. "Well, it's the only way I can save face, mother. Poor Louis. His father is always yellin' at him that as long as he lives in his house, he's gonna abide by his rules."

"Poor Louis," I commiserate.

"Whadaya mean, poor Louis? Poor Louis's father. He's askin' for it."

* * * * *

When the first copies of *If I Die At Thirty* actually arrive, we all tear open the box at once, Peggie merrily elbowing her way into position to grab the first book. Her fingers glide over the shiny jacket; she sniffs the new book smell like an ecstatic hound dog on the scent of possum.

She and I autograph copies together, Peggie always putting a smile face after her name. We think hard about what to say in Dr. Rathburn's copy. Finally I write: "With thanks for your competence and compassion." And Peggie adds: "*Ibid.* Keep yo-yo-ing. ☺"

Halloween is another gala occasion. Peg has achieved no small fame of late as a party giver, but her Halloween party is definitely her best effort, what with convicts and tigers and footed garbage bags wandering into our house, and all the sounds of hilarity whooping out.

"Do you ever wonder why you're such a happy person, Peg?"

"Well, what would you do if you had a father who gave civilization five years and a mother who was always writing books on death? I mean, sometimes I think me bein' cheery is my stubbornness acting against you guys." Just in case we might be getting swelled heads with her turning out so well.

Well, it is true that twenty years ago Joe gave the United States twenty years. Sometimes I think he's disappointed that our civilization hasn't fallen. And it's true that writing my second book, *Following Joey Home*, has been emotionally exhausting for me.

"Do you realize, mother, that you never say you're happy? Even before Joey died, I can't remember your actually sayin' you were happy. You're just depressed an awful lot of the time. Like you get these two tones in your voice I cannot stand, and one is your remind tone, and the other is your self-pity tone. Come to think of it, mother, I'm not sure you have any other tones. I mean, I try to bring you pleasure."

Shock and dismay! For so long I have done my best to be a good mother by doing all the right things for Peg, when all along the most right thing I could have done was have my own life in order.

All through the years Joe has been the one to do the fun things with Peggie. I spent so much time with the children doing things that had to be done that when Joe set out to play Scrabble with them or stamp smiley faces on their foreheads, I hid in my study to have a few minutes to myself.

Peggie's hair is finally long enough to curl, and every morning I go over it with the curling iron. As soon as she moves her head, however, the curls come out and her hair goes every which way. Tonight I suggest that we experiment, that I roll one side of her head on rollers and put the other side up on pin curls.

"Oh, could you, mother? Would you?"

As I embark on my rolling and pinning, Peg eyes me suspiciously. "Why are you doing this? Do you consider this work or fun? Fun? Oh, okay. Oh, this dumb hair. Don't I have the dumbest hair? I wonder how it will turn out. How do you think it will turn out? I feel like a washerwoman. Here I am scrubbing my clothes. Oh, I can't bend my head. Why are you doing this to me? Ow! Ow!

"Are you sure you consider this fun?"

Later when we go out for ice cream, Peggie sits straight in her chair, dips her spoon properly into her sundae, and raises it slowly to a mouth that has been gaping wide during the whole procedure. Then she makes a show of brushing off her elbows.

We are feeling silly, and we laugh until we cannot stop laughing. We laugh behind our menus; we laugh into our napkins. We laugh until we are weak laughing.

Peg picks up her napkin and with a dainty flourish tucks it into the neck of her sweater—under the back of her head. Not to be outdone, I flourish my napkin—and sit on it. We laugh until everyone in the restaurant turns and stares, until we are sick laughing.

Sometimes I get hung up on the hard time my adolescent gives me, but she gives me happy times, too. "Oh, Peggie," I choke. "When you leave, whatever will I do to manufacture my own sunshine?"

Christmas is here again. New York grandmother and grandfather are here again. We eat in the Holiday Inn and have our picture taken in front of the big red sled in the lobby again, all wearing our traditional Christmas outfits.

This year Peggie concentrates on my Christmas list as hard as on her own, keeping at me about my comparative longing for each item until she can place an appropriate number of stars after each one.

> perfume ***
> hanging plant ******
> night on the town ********
> 1.95 pen with fine point ***
> lip gloss **
> slippers, not fuzzy ****

Peg spends most of the holidays spread out on the family room floor, surrounded by charts and diagrams, working on our family tree. Memphis grandmother has always been interested in the Woodson genealogy and is glad to have someone to share her enthusiasm.

Peg wants and gets a four-drawer file cabinet for Christmas. She already has a two-drawer file cabinet but is running out of space, what with a file for every person from whom she has ever received a letter or card, a file for each of her birthdays, for every Christmas, for every school year.

I wonder about her need to preserve both past and present. Does she feel that if this is all she is to have in this life, she had best nail it down?

Peg and I go to our early Christmas Eve service so we can watch "The Nutcracker Suite" on television later on.

"I don't know why I'm developing such a love for ballet," I tell Peg, "except that beauty is important to me, and ballet is such a graceful, delicate kind of beauty."

"Yeah, it reminds me of figure skating at the Olympics or somebody playin' the harp. It's good to be able to admire the human body."

When I look over at Peg toward the end of the performance,

she is weeping away in what is obviously a noisy process on the inside but as silent as this silent night on the outside. "You weren't supposed to see me crying unless you were crying," she gulps, smearing her cheeks with her fists. "I don't know what's the matter with me. It's just that Clara doesn't want to leave her dream, but she has to. She has to go back to the playroom, and, oh, mother, she loses her prince."

I happen to pass by Peg's room toward the end of Christmas week when she is displaying her new file cabinet to Denise. "Now don't forget, Denise," I hear her say, "when I die, it's your responsibility to give each of our friends the folder with his or her name on it."

* * * * *

Somewhere I hear that one of the best ways parents can pass their faith along to their children is by sharing with them some of their own inner spiritual happenings. True, our children absorb a lot of what we are osmotically, but a lot that we think and feel they can't absorb because they can't sense that it's there.

I wait till Peg and I have a cozy moment and then relate to her an experience I had way back when she was a baby. She likes stories about when she was little. "We were driving home from a day of fishing on the Tennessee River, Peg. I was tired, and you were fussing in the back seat.

"I had my head half out the window trying to cool off when I happened to look up at the most radiant sunset I had ever seen. The sky was dark, kind of a black-blue, and velvet ribbons of pink and baby blue rippled across it, shaded so daintily and fading so rapidly that I felt I could not bear the loss."

Peg listens with her open face.

"I had the strongest feeling that if I had been the only person on earth, God still would have painted that sunset as a response to something He saw of worth in me, something about me He found lovable. And as soon as I truly believed that God found me lovable, I found lovable a woman I'd never been able to stand before—the meanest woman in our church."

I don't describe my sky as though I expect Peggie to be affected by it, but only as something I want her to know because it has affected me.

When I'm through, Peg goes off and makes a sign on blue construction paper with rose crayon. *Smile—God finds you lovable* it reads, with a big smile face on the side. "This is for you, mother," she says, presenting the sign to me ceremoniously.

But after a while she takes it back and hangs it on the door of her room.

* * * * *

I decide that if I am going to share some of my spiritual successes with Peggie, I should let her in on some of my fiascos, too. I search my memories for a failure, however slight, to which she might relate.

"Remember that time you were in the hospital and Tom Rader was in, too?" I ask, referring to a counselor from C.F. Camp who had had C.F. himself and who had died recently. "Well, one day I was walking by his room, and he looked out and smiled at me, and I knew he was inviting me in. But I never felt comfortable with young men his age, especially young men with ponytails, so I made believe I didn't see him and walked by. I've always been sorry about that."

"Oh, mother, really? That makes me feel good to know you did something like that."

For all her insults, does Peg regard Joe and me more highly than we think? Perhaps she feels herself insulted by what she views as our maturity or even our perfection. She does not respect me less when I admit to fallibility, but, less threatened perhaps, is able to respect me more.

"I'll never be as good as you are," Peg laments on occasion.

"Oh, Peg, in a lot of ways you're way ahead of me. You're miles ahead of where I was when I was your age. Your spirit takes time to grow just as your body does. Let me show you this quote from my C. S. Lewis calendar:

Good and evil both increase at compound interest. That is why the little decisions you and I make every day are of such infinite importance. The smallest good act today is the capture of a strategic point from which, a few months later, you may be able to go on to victories you never dreamed of.

"Well, I don't know what you expect me to do, but I'm sure not gonna scribble that down on a napkin. I mean, you always do this to me. You read a poem or something that means a lot to you, and then you look at me like I'm gonna say it's wonderful, and I don't see what it's talking about, and you get upset with me because you want me to see it so badly.

"And you're always telling me what communion means to

you. Do you ever stop to think how that makes a kid feel who doesn't get anything out of communion?"

I explain what I think the quote is about.

"Oh, well, now I understand. But I'm still not gonna scribble it down on a napkin."

*   *   *   *   *

Patti, Peg's best friend from C.F. Camp, is in the hospital, and Peg and I go to visit. I wouldn't have taken Peg, though, if I'd known Patti would be lying there, a bag of bones, as they say, an oxygen mask strapped to her face, looking as though she did not have the strength even to lie in a hospital bed.

Patti's mother and I go down to the cafeteria, but Patti grabs Peggie's hand. "Don't go, Peggie. Stay with me, Peggie." I don't know what the girls talk about, but Peg sags when the visit is over and we walk down the hall.

She's standing beside me a few days later when the call from Patti's mother comes.

"Did Patti die, mother?"

"Yes, honey."

"Everybody I know with C.F. is dead." Peg turns an awesome wrath on me. "I'll tell you one thing. I will never go to C.F. Camp again, not without Joey and not without Patti. Oh, mother, I'll miss her."

The next week Joe and I are in the family room when Peg storms in and slams her books on the floor. "Do you really think they speak French in heaven?" she demands. "And precisely how will I use algebra when I'm in the hospital all the time?"

She squeezes in between Joe and me on the couch. "And what about college? Should I go or not? I mean, there'd be so little time left to do anything."

Joe tells Peg that if she thinks she might like to move to the inner city after high school and teach people to read or some such thing, that that's an option she should consider. But he warns her that she better not absolutely plan on dying in case that isn't God's plan.

"Sometimes when I can't get my French, and Madame is yelling at me, I think about how God knows not only English and French but every language in the whole world. It helps me feel how big He is."

Joe emphasizes that the one thing people take with them when they die is what they've learned. "People who know they may not have long to live have more reason than most to keep on *becoming*, Peg. I hope you'll take your love of living with you whenever you die."

"And my love of eating, father? Should I keep that goin' good, too?" Peg winks at me. "Mangeons dans un restaurant ce soir, papa?"

*   *   *   *   *

Would you mind if I tore off the cover of this magazine to hang in my room?" Peg asks. A picture of a large hand cradling the globe dominates the cover along with a verse from Isaiah: "Is it for you to question me about my children and to dictate to me what my hands should do? It was I who made the earth, and created man who is on it."

"Remember how you told me once, mother, about when we were in Tennessee and daddy was trying to find a new church, and he looked and looked all over the South and couldn't find one? And then we heard about the C.F. Center here and it bein' the best and all, and right off three churches around Cleveland wanted him? Well, I been thinkin' about that. That seems like some kind of sign to me."

I know what kind of sign Peg means. Joey is dead, and Patti is dead, and last night she could not sleep for coughing, but God knows we're here. He cares.

Every once in a while Peg asks if we can have some of the conversations we had about death when she was thirteen* over again, especially the one about why bad things happen to people, but somehow we never get around to it. The year when Peggie was thirteen and learned that "kids with C.F. might die young" was the year to talk about death. This year when she is fifteen is the year for Peggie to live with the death of one kid brother with C.F. and not need to talk about it.

She is comforted by the control she feels God has over every event in a person's life; she is also careful about the control she feels every person has over his or her own life. I talk to her about theological paradoxes, but Peg is not interested in abstractions.

"What I would really like to know, mother, is this: Do you think daddy will drive more carefully now that he knows deep down he doesn't have permanent safety?"

* * * * *

*See footnote on page 42.

Some time ago Peg entered a state-wide English competition. Today she gets the word. She came in eleventh in the state.

"Too bad it couldn't have been tenth," Judy commiserates.

But Peggie doesn't mind. "How could it be, mother? Me, eleventh out of all the best English students in Ohio? Me, who's never best in anything? Me, eleventh out of 40,000 kids? Did you pray about it, mother?"

"Actually, Peggie, I don't think you should be so surprised. You're gifted in English. But to answer your question, yes, I did ask God that you would do the best you were capable of doing."

"Boy, that sure was nice of Him," Peg gurgles. "Ya know, there's this one thing about school I don't like, mother, and that's that so many of the kids are burnouts, and they never get excited about anything."

The first thing I must understand about burnouts is that not all the kids are burnouts, she takes time to explain. A lot of the kids are really fun. Some of the nice kids think they have to act like burnouts, but they're nice anyway. Real burnouts are kids who come to school and do nothing but sit, if they come to school at all.

"You look in their eyes and it's like they're vacant, like there's no thinkin' behind them. It's so sad when you look in a burnout's eyes, mother, like everything inside their head's been burned out."

Peg looks shyly into my eyes. "You want to know the real difference between me and a burnout? Well, a burnout doesn't want nothin', nothin' at all. But me, because I'm a Christian, ya know—I want to be like Jesus." She darts from the room, grabbing her latest *Campus Life* as she goes. "Forget I ever said that," she calls back. "Boy, did that ever sound pious."

Then she streaks back into the kitchen, her magazine unfurled over her head. "My book! *If I Die at Thirty!* They have a review of my book!" She sits at the table sheltering the page with her arms. No way may I peek at the review till she has read every word.

"They like it! They think it's really good! But listen to this: 'The book does leave some questions unanswered. Is Peggie Woodson still alive?'"

Peggie dashes to her typewriter. "Campus Life:" she taps. "Dear Sirs: I am Peggie Woodson and I am STILL ALIVE."

Sixteen Years Old

Peggie preserves her sixteenth birthday in her diary, every detail notable.

March 14

Mother says I should write in my diary about the events of my sixteenth birthday! I guess I should be non-original and start at the beginning.

Lots of mysterious things happened in the last week (odd talks between Derrick and Denise, etc.) but they were explained because we were all going ice-skating on Friday night, and they were all going to bring me presents at the rink. I worried all day before Mary was to pick me up about how embarrassed I was going to be at the skating rink. Mary picked me up. She said that they had just been shopping and they still had to get her skates. I swollowed it like a dummy! She asked me if I would bring her packages in and put them in the family room while she went to get her skates. I had my suspitions, but it was so reasonable! I opened the door to the family room and they all yelled surprise!

We opened presents. Louis—blue butterfly earrings with 14K gold posts; Lester—a candle and make-them-yourself smiley face stickers; Judy—earring tree; Glad—bird stationary—"Happiness is something to sing about"; John—picture (Faith is the substance of things hoped for, the evidence of things not seen"—St. Paul). John and Glad gave me the same card—B.C. playing a clarinet.

Mary gave me 16 sugar cubes which I have to keep till I'm 17. All of her cups, plates, and tablecloth matched. Mary had gone to my house when I wasn't home and asked my mother for some enzymes so I could eat at the party—sneaky, sneaky!

We played Ooga Boog. We also played a game with toothpicks and lifesavers. Stand in two lines, everyone has a toothpick in their mouth. You had to pass the lifesaver forward and back. I called mother and asked her to bring up her camera.

Today Becky and Mrs. K. took me out to eat at a buffet—can't spell "smorgasborg?" At church Aunt Kate and Uncle Jim gave me a totem pole plant. I put my 16 pennies in the sunday school bank and got a pin and a pencil. hee hee My birthday this year—sweet 16—will certainly be a remembered joy that will never be past!

* * * * *

Boy, my favorite day again. Guess I have to sit in church with you again."

"Is that so bad?"

"You don't talk to me. You don't want me to talk to you. Sitting with you is like sitting with nobody."

Peg proceeds with her denunciation of church nonstop all the way to church. "And you can't turn off the sermon like you can turn off the TV if it gets boring. You just have to sit there, and you can't do anything else like sketch at the same time. You can't move. I think it would be a good idea to at least take notes.

"Even in Sunday school, which is nice, you hear the same stuff over and over. Like Eve always has a lamb in front of her, and mothers are always baking pies. I like the teacher we have now, 'cause she makes you think."

Peg pursues her diatribe of church with renewed vigor all the way home from church. "Remember when you were tellin' me out of the catechism that time about glorifying God and enjoying Him forever? Well, I was really surprised about the enjoying part. I never thought about enjoying God, 'cause I sure never enjoyed church."

Until recently we had two sessions of Sunday school, one before and one during adult worship. Peg went to early Sunday school as a student and to second Sunday school as a teacher, and she loved and learned from both. Now we only have Sunday school after church, and Peg cannot escape "those old hymns and all that stuff in the sermons I hear at home."

On conversation day in French recently the kids matched each other with various occupations. Who would make the best minister? Gladie. The best judge? Peggie.

"Still," I lament to Joe, "it's not Peggie's sin, but ours, if Peggie's bored in church."

"I have homework to do this afternoon," Peg raves on, "but I know I won't be able to do my homework. Ya wanna know how I know I won't be able to do my homework? Because every Sunday my mind gets so turned off, it's Monday before I can get it turned back on."

I splurge. It takes all morning and afternoon, but I find just the pantsuit and purse and shoes to give me that I'm-going-to-a-writers'-conference-*as-a-speaker* look. "Do something daring with my hair," I tell them at the beauty shop.

"Well, what do you think, Peg?" I model the new, chic me with a hesitance as old as my own adolescence.

Peg thinks the pantsuit makes my hips look big. My hair is okay—if I don't mind lookin' like every other middle-aged woman. She gawks at my shoes and giggles. *"You're* gonna wear *them?"*

Peggie outdoes herself in snitiness these days. "Will you be home tonight, Peg?" I ask. "Yeah, another night with you, another night shot." She slams out of the car whenever I take her someplace, not saying thank you, not saying good-bye.

It's strange, but almost all I can give form to on paper, or in my mind, are the nice times we have together, but mostly I *feel* the nasty times.

I explain to Peg that I value her opinion and that her ridicule hurts. But she scoffs at every effort I make to understand what is hurting her. "What would you know, mother? How would you understand?"

Today I reach my limit. I can give form to today.

"Okay, Peggie, that is enough. I will not take one more fresh-mouth comment from you. Not one more, do you understand? I am still the mother around here. If you can't say something human to me, don't say anything at all."

"I can't help it if your hair looks like the gerbils' nest!"

I clout her in the mouth. Peace-loving me. I plunge up the stairs and down into the soft solace of my bed, my pillow moist. What Peg is doing I do not care. There is no hope for us.

We sit in the family room after supper, unwilling parties to an uneasy truce. "This project I'm workin' on for English is coming pretty good," she mutters. "Even if I have been working on it by myself all week."

"Why by yourself?"

"Well, the teacher told us to go in groups of three, and John went with Mary and Denise, and Judy and Derrick and Louis went together, and nobody was left for me.''

So she's been rejected again, and that's why she's been especially intent on rejecting me. So okay. Some rejection is a part of everybody's life.

So she doesn't like being dependent on my taking her places. We'll let her drive herself as soon as she's able, but right now she is dependent on me. And much as adolescents need to put distance of every kind between themselves and their parents, some evenings Peg will have to spend in the same room with me.

So it's a difficult time of life for her. I will still call the limits. I will absorb so much of her wrath, if that will help her, but so much and no more. What am I teaching Peg about how to handle injury when I let her heap insult upon insult on me?

We parents of adolescents are going through a difficult time of life, too.

*   *   *   *   *

Come here, mother. I have to show you something," Peg yells, besieging the front door.

It is the grass, calf-high and a just-fertilized green. "Have you ever seen anything so pretty? I mean, look at all those other cropped lawns cut so close. They're not nearly so pretty, but look at ours. How tall that grass must be, six or seven inches, I bet, and so bright. It looks just like the grass in an Easter basket, doesn't it, mother? Look at it blowin' in the breeze."

Later when she glances out the window and sees her father plowing paths of desolation through her beautiful field, she charges outside and plants herself in front of him, waving her arms in the manner of a policeman stopping traffic at a busy intersection, berating Joe over the roar of the mower.

She refuses an Easter basket this year. "All the little kids in Sunday school think about is the Easter bunny," she explains. "You say, 'What does Easter mean to you?' and they jump up and down shouting, 'The Easter bunny. The Easter bunny.'" But Peg has her Easter-basket grass.

"You do think the birds will nest in our chimney again this year, don't you, mother? I mean, I can't wait to hear those faint peep-peeps every spring, and then they chirp louder, and then they sing along with the music on the TV."

Peg finds uncommon beauty in unlikely places, and woe to anyone who defiles it. "You guys didn't actually build a fire in the fireplace this winter, did you? Like burning up the nest when I wasn't around? *Did you?* DID YOU, father? Mother, DID *YOU?*"

* * * * *

I decide to tell Peg how pleased I am at the good job she's doing of picking up her books. Her sweaters. The popsicle sticks from her Sunday school craft project. But if I once found it hard to squelch words of disapproval, I now find it hard to speak words of praise. Is this another of my negative reactions to my teenager's negative reactions to me? Or was the order of our mutual contrariness reversed? Which came first, my mother chicken pecking or her hard-boiled eggishness?

I know I complimented Peg lavishly when she was little, but now I keep putting off this simplest of thank yous, waiting for the right opportunity. Finally I blurt it out.

"Why are you doing this to me, mother?"

I explain that mothers often keep yelling at their children about areas in which they need to change, but see no point in mentioning areas that don't need improvement. But that this is defeating, because if parents comment only when their kids are bad, kids come to think of themselves as only bad, and it gets harder and harder for them to be good.

"Yeah, like there's this one teacher who's out to ruin my whole life. If you ask a question, she yells what kind of education have you had that you don't know anything. Don't you ever read? How could you be so dumb? But if you don't ask questions, she yells don't you have any curiosity? Don't you want to learn? I get so depressed in that class. Sometimes I think I can't stand it if she yells one more time, and sometimes I feel like yelling back."

"Well, I just want to be sure you understand how much it means when you put away your records and your mail and your gloves and your candle-making equipment. It's a big help to me."

"Well, you do good things, too, ya know. You clean good, and you write good, and you cook good, and you dress good."

When I recover, I tell Peg that I'm going to make a point of complimenting her more often, but never unless I really mean it.

"And you always drive me places, and you give me reasonable curfews. And you don't make me wear clothes I don't like, though sometimes you try to persuade hard. And you let me have kids over, and you go upstairs and don't embarrass me. I mean, I can be pretty sure you're not gonna do anything dumb. And you buy Cokes for my friends. You help me, too, ya know."

* * * * *

Ya know how father's always talkin' about the peace and joy of Christ in his heart? And you're always sayin' the presence of God means so much to you? Well, I can't say anything like that. I can't even say Jesus is my friend, 'cause a friend talks back, and Jesus never talks back to me.

"I mean, all the kids who go to The Living Room—ya know, that's the Christian Coffeehouse—are always saying, 'Jesus came into my life on the 8th of May at 3:15 in the afternoon,' and they all think it has to happen to you like that. Me and Becky are the only ones who can't remember a time.

"And I know you say sometimes it happens gradually, but if it happens that way, how can you be sure it happened? Like everybody always says they had an emptiness within, but I don't feel an emptiness. Sometimes when my friends aren't around and I feel real lonely, I wonder if that's what they're talkin' about.

"I mean, I don't know any way of knowing if God's there except for Him to go away, and I'd feel the emptiness, and then He could come back, and I would know He was there, but I don't want Him to go away to find out.

"I asked this kid at The Living Room once—wasn't he glad he could feel the contrast between bein' a Christian and not, but he said no, 'cause you always remember the bad times, and you wonder how life could have been like that.

"I was readin' this book the other day, and the author was sayin' that God can't come into your heart through a closed door, and that sometimes you have a besetting sin in your life that keeps the door of your heart closed. He sure did use funny language. You don't think I have a besetting sin, do you? Oh, no. I hope not. What could my closed door be?"

Later she scrawls solemnly away on a slip of smiley-face pad paper and files it away in her tenth-grade folder.

Why am I so lonely? I keep looking for a kindred spirit, but I will never find a true one because I am an individual. No one has my personality but me. At best I can hope to find, in other people, parts of what would be my kindred spirit. No one person will ever understand me fully—except Jesus—but it is so much harder to talk to him than to a friend. But if I reach out and really make the effort, maybe I can combine all of those different elements in different people.

Jesus may be harder to talk to personally, but he can speak in indirect ways. I have never in my life talked to Maxi for 1½ hours at one time—and I enjoyed it besides.

Jesus really had this problem. He would have even more trouble finding anything resembling a kindred spirit because, even tho human, he was so pure and knew and understood so much more than those he associated with.

* * * * *

Our church's Women's Fellowship asks Peggie and me to have the program for their mother-daughter banquet. We rummage through our memory box and decide to put on a skit entitled "Mother's Day Cards Through the Years." My favorite card consists of a poem Peggie made up on her way home from school one day when she was ten.

I had a whim
Just to begin
My mothers day poem today
So don't get mad
Just stay real glad
That I have come your way.

Your hair's sometimes a mess
But you usually say yes
Whenever I ask a favor
You have whacked once or twice
Though you're really quite nice
It's you I savor.

We're not real rich
But we're not in a ditch
You never drink a boo*
You're not the God of Mammon
But we can afford salmon
I'll never be poor with you.

You're full of fire
You have a great sire
That must be why you're great
You don't sniff glue
You're really true
You have a nice mate.

When I get through
If I ever do
I hope you like my note
You're really smart
With a big place in my heart
On you I dote.

*boos—drinks (like beer)
  a boo—one drink

I guess it's my favorite card because it represents what I've come to feel are the happiest years of a mother's life, those elementary school years when your children are old enough to do things for themselves but are still emotionally dependent on you. Still young enough to believe you are "full of fire" and "great" and "smart" and "nice" and "true."

Older friends tell me that if you hang in there long enough with your teenagers—keep loving them, don't retaliate with unkindness for unkindness, hold the lines of communication open—they come back. That your best years are the years when you relate to your children as adults.

My mind tells me they may be right, but my heart cries no. There will never be a time when Peggie will dote on me quite as she doted on me when she skipped and scribbled her way home from school that proud, elaborate day when she was ten. And no years will ever be as good as those years when Peggie doted on me.

* * * * *

Everybody's finding boyfriends and jobs," wails Peg. "I'm not gonna have anybody to do anything with this summer."

Judy, it seems, has had the same boyfriend for ages now. She sees him in the library in fourth period every day and walks to fifth like she's in a trance. And all the boys like Mary. And Denise is so silly. She likes somebody different every week.

"I don't see what this fuss about boys is all about. It only means trouble. You wouldn't believe all these soap operas I'm in the middle of, mother. One person likes another person, who doesn't like them back. Two people like each other, and then one of them changes their mind. Somebody's always crying.

"And Gladie's in this ecology club, and she's always telling us the earth is being destroyed, and she's so hyper about it. And Becky says every time she sprays under her arms she thinks she's destroying the ozone layer.

"Do you think I could get a job, mother? Now why am I crying? Isn't that the dumbest thing?"

Peggie decides that before she goes outside to look for summer work, she'll look for typing she can do at home. She puts an ad in the *Cleveland Press. Home Typing of all kinds. Electric typewriter. Peggie Woodson. 845-4281.*

The phone rings once. "It's for you, Peg—a man," I whisper.

Peggie springs on the phone like a lioness on a lamb with whom she has not yet learned to lie down together. Then she purrs into the lamb's ear. "This is Peggie Woodson. . . . Why, yes. Yes, I would be!" She cannot keep the lilt from her lady voice. But suddenly her tone changes. "I'm not interested in that. . . . No, thank you for calling, but I am not interested. . . . I AM NOT INTERESTED."

"He kept offering me more and more money to type envelopes for pornography, as if I would do that for any amount of money. Boy, there's a lot of sick people out there, mother."

Finally I hire Peggie as my secretary. I need a secretary, and she is a good one, but typing for her mother is not the kind of job Peggie needs.

She applies at the library. She applies at two bookstores, scattering notes around both the upstairs and downstairs phones.

Hello, my name is Peggie Woodson, and I was wondering if you need any part-time help, either permanently or just for the summer.

Yes	No
when would it be conv. for me to come in for an interview?	would it do me any good to fill out an app. for sometime in the future?

She fills out applications and hopes again beside a phone "that must be out of order, mother." She applies at a steakhouse, trying on three outfits in preparation for the interview. Mary and Derrick and Lester and a whole other bunch of kids at school have jobs at this steakhouse.

"I think I did pretty good," she reports. "I mean, I was really mature. I told them I would work on Sundays in emergencies when they really needed me, but that I wouldn't work during church time. I had to say if I had any health condition that would affect my work, and I didn't think C.F. would, but I thought I'd be honest and put it down anyway. The manager's gonna call me in three days if he wants me."

For five days I am not permitted to leave the house.

"If God thinks it's good for me to get this job, I'll get it, because if it's important to Him, I'll get it, and what's good for me is important to Him, right?"

"Well, of course you have to commit it to Him."

"Well, of course it's committed to Him. Whadaya think? Okay, now just so you'll know, from now on everything in my life is committed to Him."

"No phone call, right?" she asks as she plods in from her wanderings on the fifth day.

"Daddy's not coming home tonight, Peg. How about going shopping for a new top and eating out?"

"What do you think, mother? Why everybody else and not me?" Peg drags by my side through The May Co. department store.

"Well, I hate to say this, honey, but given a healthy person and a person with a strange-sounding disease, a lot of employers are going to choose the healthy person. Then, too, customers might not like having a hostess who coughs on their food. You may have to work harder than most kids to find the right job."

"Nobody looks at me weird in school any more when I cough. Everybody that doesn't know I have C.F. thinks it's smoker's cough. Isn't that neat?" Peg gives a little bob just thinking about the kids thinking she has smoker's cough. "I mean, I go into one of my coughing fits and perfectly strange kids tell me I better lay off the cigarettes!"

But soon she is sober again. "You don't think it's my skinny arms or my black teeth, do you, mother?"

"Your arms aren't that skinny any more, Peg." I pull her inside the ladies' room and stand her in front of me before the mirror, draping my arms over her shoulders. "Now whose arms would you rather have, your slightly skinny arms or my enormously flabby arms?" We spend five hysterical minutes in The May Co. ladies' room trying our arms on each other before a customer comes in intent on more basic pursuits.

Peg looks at me curiously as we stroll back through the store. "How can I be an adult, mother, when I have no model?"

* * * * *

The day Peg goes for her driver's test actually arrives—the most worried-about, waited-for of all her days. Joe takes her to a testing station an hour on the east side of Cleveland to avoid Big Mama—Big Mama being one of the testers at the west side station. Peggie has it on the best authority that if you get Big Mama, you are doomed before you get behind the wheel.

She talked us into letting her take driver's ed at a private school shortly after she turned sixteen so she wouldn't have to wait till fall to take it at high school, and she came home daily with accounts of the advances the men instructors made to the girl students when they had them alone in the cars. I was entrusted with these naughty newscasts only after I'd crossed my heart and hoped for five publisher's rejections in a row if I told father. Father, she was sure, would jerk her right out of driving school if he knew.

Then a woman instructor was assigned to Peg. So what if she spent most of her driving time chauffeuring the instructor's boyfriend to work? She had to drive someplace, didn't she? "It does seem strange, though, that we always pick him up at her place, mother. I don't know what's goin' on there. And she has this big picture of a naked woman on her refrigerator. What would anybody want to do that for?"

Somehow with all the transporting of the boyfriend, the instructor never gets around to parallel parking, and Mr. Anderson, Peg's beloved Sunday school superintendent for as long as she can remember, spends hours teaching her to parallel park. "Isn't that nice of him? Isn't he the sweetest man, mother?"

The whole thing appears to be a lark for Peg, especially having her own set of keys—green keys for the green car, blue keys for the blue car. She gets her own house key at the same time, the house, unfortunately, being black and white. Did we think we could paint the shutters red? No? Well, she'd get a red key for the house anyway.

So what if she can't see out the windshield without sitting on a cushion? I'm hunting all over town for a blue car cushion and a green car cushion, right?

The only thing that annoys her are neighbors and church members gaping as she chugs down the block or up the church drive. "What? Are you old enough to drive, Peggie?"

I keep wanting to remind her that driving is a deadly serious business, but I get in enough trouble soundlessly hitting the floor with my brake foot as I ride beside her.

Then she confides in me before she leaves for her test that she has promised herself she will never drive without her seat belt fastened or go faster than the speed limit or break any other law, and that so far she has not done so. Once she did forget to put her blinker on before she moved into the next lane, but she put it on real quick after she got there to help her remember the next time, so that infraction didn't count.

She comes home waving her driver's license in a triumphant arc over her head. Even her picture came out good. Her hair is longer now, and she wears it parted in the middle and tied together under each ear with an elastic band. "I asked them if approximate was all right for my weight, and they said it was, so I said *ninety*."

The letters on our license plates this year are MA. Peggie says they stand for Margaret Ann, her real name. Joe says they're the car's way of hollering for help when she takes the corners on two wheels.

*   *   *   *   *

Peggie and her Bible are of one piece, its denim cover blending with her blue jeans, her blond hair trailing its pages as she curls up around it on the living room couch surrounded by the paraphernalia of earnest research.

"You know how I can't stand just reading the Bible, mother? Well, father has this book where you can look up a Bible verse on a subject, and it tells you where other verses on the subject are. I'm lookin' up all the verses I can find on *light.*

"Like there's this verse that says one of the names for God is Father of Lights. I never knew that. Isn't that cheery? Doesn't that remind you of smile faces? And then another verse says we're children of light. And that parallel is all through, like Jesus is the Light of the World, and we're the light of the world. Isn't that the most interesting thing?

"Now reading the Bible that way's not so bad, is it, mom?"

I know what you're doing, Peg, polishing your ideals, removing the tarnish they acquired when they ventured out of their protective home covers and into the worlds of job hunting and driving school.

I gave Peggie a book of daily Bible selections for teenagers once, but she kept forgetting to read it. I suggested that she keep it in the bathroom, where she'd be sure to have a few uninterrupted minutes to give it every day, and she thought that was a good idea. "Like you keep Dietrich Bonhoeffer in the bathroom, right, mother?" But she never brought the book in there.

I'm glad I didn't push the Bible reading. It's good to see Peggie discovering the Bible now, not only in her own way to meet her own need, but in her own time and of her own volition.

"If you ever do write another book about me, mother, I hope you put in about Pete and Dolores's Bible studies. I mean, Pete asks us questions on contemporary issues, and we get in these terrible arguments, and we try to defend ourselves with the Bible. That's why I like youth group so much.

"Though I must admit that last week we all went on strike in the hall and refused to go in till Pete agreed we didn't have to pray out loud. Ya know, goin' around in a circle, wondering what you're going to say when it's your turn. You don't have to put in the book that I was the instigator of that.

"Do you ever wonder if anybody's really up there when you pray, mother?"

"I used to."

"Well, sometimes I start praying, and then this other me starts questioning the me that's praying. 'How are you going to feel if you find out someday that nobody's up there? Won't you feel stupid talkin' to empty air?' And then this other me answers back with how I know somebody's there, and I end up with three of me talkin' at once.

"Do you think God gets bored with long prayers? I mean, you can tell if people mean it or if they just say the words. I spend a lot of time apologizing when I pray, 'cause I don't want to go on and on. 'I hate to do this, God,' I say, 'but I'm going to sleep.'

"Or right in the middle of praying, I get into a big thought, and then I realize I'm in the middle of praying, and I apologize for forgetting. I mean, I apologize real fast. 'Sorry about that, God,' I say. And then I think, 'This is really dumb telling God I'm sorry I forgot I was praying to Him.'"

Well, however immature or mature Peggie's prayers may be, when Peggie Woodson talks to God, that's Peggie Woodson talking. I'm glad Joe and I haven't pressed her into acting out any form of piety not natural to her stage of development. If we had, now when she's rebelling against us, would she be rebelling against what was really our piety as well?

"I'll tell ya one thing I'm sure God gets bored with, mother, and that's people thankin' Him three times a day for their food. I bet He tunes you guys right out when you do that."

* * * * *

Peggie's advanced English friends play baseball up at the high school during their spare time this summer. Peg dons her red shorts and red and blue striped top and manages to bike herself up there. She doesn't have the strength to hit or run, however, and after several humiliating attempts, she decides to be water boy—or, more accurately, Kool-Aid girl. "This way I'm popular, mother."

I buy her a set of plastic cups and a thermos.

"Did I tell you about the other night when we were drivin' to that party, and Lester called 'Chinese fire drill' and jumped out of the car and ran around it? Oh, mother, you wouldn't believe how much fun we had.

"And then at the party when we ran out of stuff to do, everybody decided to go out in the yard and play stickball, and I didn't want to go, but they made me, and both captains chose me first for their teams. And the team that got me were all jumpin' up and down shouting, 'We got her! We got her!'

"The police were watching us the other day up at the school. I don't think too many kids our age get together to play baseball. Gladie says, 'Oh, I think it's so wonderful that we can all be together like this.'"

Well, I think it's wonderful, too. Peggie's ninth-grade lifeboat friends float high and ever fiercely loyal in the vaster seas of senior high.

"Ya know, there's this one thing Gladie can't stand, and that's how now and then one of her ears sticks through her hair. You want to know what I say when one of them peeks through? I say, 'Hi, ear.' You wouldn't believe the conversations I have with one or another of Gladie's ears. 'Haven't seen you in quite a while, ear.' Poor Glad." Peg laughs with her whole face, both arms, and the lower part of her left leg.

Peg is always finding something to laugh almost-all-over about, even Becky fainting in the movies. When Joe and the girls get to the theater, a crowd is waiting to get in, and Becky keeps saying she's going to faint. Joe and Peg ignore her because, they say, I am always threatening to faint and never doing it. But Becky does it. She faints flat away in the lobby of the theater.

"You know what?" Peggie chortles. "It really is true that you fall forward when you faint. We were a bigger sensation than 'That Darn Cat.'"

When she goes home with Becky to help her babysit, Peg and Becky's brother tell the child they have Becky shut up in a bottle. Then they make whatever is in the bottle go up in smoke. "I don't know when I've had so much fun," Peg screams into the phone. "Can I sleep over?"

She's grown so much through loneliness and pain; now I pray she will find God also through friendship and laughter. That she and Becky will look up from their sleeping bags giggling and find Him standing there.

* * * * *

Peggie has a job. Just Saturday mornings and two afternoons a week, but in an office! For minimum wage!

"I sure do like my job," she trills to Joe as she waltzes into the house after her first day at work. "It gets a little boring filing all morning, but you know me and how I like to organize things.

"Ya know how Mary says the manager at the steakhouse is always bragging about how many girls he made cry that day? Well, Mr. Peabody kept tellin' me what a good worker I was, and I heard him telling his partner how he kept suggesting I take breaks, but I wouldn't take breaks, and what a good little worker I was. I mean, I really do try to be a good worker."

I listen from behind the closed door of my study. Joe isn't often home when Peg bursts in to recount her happenings, and it's only right that he should have this big telling to himself.

"And working for my neighbor is great—he understands about C.F. and all, and if I have to go in the hospital, he won't fire me, and I can catch up on the filing later. They're gonna teach me how to do insurance policies, too, and in the fall I'm gonna keep on workin' part-time after school.

"Will it be all right with you, father, if I buy a little TV for my room if I'm payin' for it with my own money? Like I could watch 'Star Trek' while you're watching the news and all. I think instead of giving God 10 percent of my paycheck, I'm gonna give Him 11 percent so I'll be doing more than I'm supposed to."

I peek out of my study in time to see Joe give Peggie a big hug, his face shining with fatherly pride.

"Ya know, I think this is the best job I could have gotten. Do you suppose God knew if I waited I'd get this one, and that's why I didn't get the others?"

* * * * *

Infection has been building up in Peg's lungs, and Dr. Rathburn puts her in the hospital to get her lungs cleaned out before school starts.

"You know how sometimes married people need to take a vacation from each other?" Peg asks the minute we are alone in her room following admission procedures. "Well, I know how you and daddy hate to make the trip across town, and I just wanna say that you don't have to come to see me unless you really, really want to. I mean, you can leave now if you have something you need to do."

I cannot believe it. Peggie's complaint has always been that I haven't come to see her often enough in the hospital, or that I've left too soon. But her present message comes through all too clearly as the days pass, the quietness of the house unbroken by what was once the eager ringing of the phone and Peg's excited prattle.

I call her on occasion. On rarer occasion I locate her. But on no occasion could our conversations be described as nourishing.

"Hi, honey," I say cheerily.

"Whadaya want?" she answers churlishly. "I was playin' cards with Alex. You always interrupt me, mother. Alex is an artist. Alex thinks I have talent."

"Well, I just wondered what you were doing."

"I told ya. I'm playing cards with Alex. So whadaya want?"

It is after one such phone call that I become ill, weak and aching all over.

If my subconscious has arranged my illness to make Peggie feel sorry for me, Peggie does not cooperate with my subconscious. "I find it highly coincidental, mother, that you should *get sick* every time I leave home. I'll be leavin' for good soon, ya know, and you better not make me feel guilty by having a nervous breakdown."

"I found her in Alex's room," Joe reports grimly, returning from a visit. Joe is accustomed to hospital visitation; he is also less easily intimidated than I. "She lives in Alex's room, Meg. He's a man, twenty-three, with long blond hair and a guitar leaning against his bed—an anti-establishment guitar, if I ever saw one."

My dizziness and sundry pains persist. I long for the time when Peggie's pleasure in anything that happened when she was away from me found completion only when she shared it with me. Now she talks to me only if she wants something.

Is this why you started every day of your life for five years with a thermometer in your mouth? I rage to myself. Is this why you lavished your energy and time and money and love for sixteen years on her welfare—so she could airily wave good-bye to you and trot off with Alexander? So she could stop being your person . . . and become her own person?

Of course, as soon as I ask the question, I know the answer. But what a blow. And how incredible that in all my awareness of my motherhood I never fully faced that critical question or that unquestionable answer.

When, after three weeks of no communication, I go to bring Peggie home from the hospital, I find her fastened to the foot of the bed of the young blond god. "We'd like to have a few more minutes, mother, if you don't mind."

I wait in the hall.

She jabbers briefly in the car on the way home. "I weigh ninety-three, mother. Can you imagine? And I made friends with this new girl. Her name is Lacey, and she has this colored TV we all watched the John Denver special on. I think she'll be one of my good C.F. friends. She's really sick, though, mother."

But soon Peg runs down. "If you don't mind not talking, mother, I have a decision concerning Alex I have to think about. You wouldn't understand. It's a very important decision, but . . . I have to make it . . . by myself."

Can all of this be as hard on her as it is on me?

*　*　*　*　*

Peggie's precious group of friends turn on her at school, accusing her of telling on one of them for cheating and then cheating herself. Neither charge is true, Peg insists, but everybody yelled at her at lunch and separated themselves from her. She cried. Finally she had to leave and go to the library.

After waiting so long for her hair to grow, Peg had it cut in a wedge in preparation for the beginning of eleventh grade. It looks darling, but at the moment the lack of those six-and-a-half inches of flaxen locks, which I rescued from the floor at Mademoiselles, adds to her air of defenselessness, and my heart cries with her.

"Let's not use that same old book," she urges her father at family discussion. "Open to Proverbs, daddy, and stick your finger in."

"The Bible is not a book of magic, Peggie."

"Oh, please, father."

Joe tells her about the man who opened the Bible and stuck a pin in to find a verse to cure his depression. The verse said, "Judas went out and hung himself."

"Come on, father. Just this once. Just for fun."

Joe opens the Bible, sticks his finger in blindly, and reads, "The wounds of a friend are sweeter than the kisses of an enemy."

I will never forget the look on Peg's face. Such wonder.

"Now don't go basing your life on things like that," I warn her.

"I know, mother. I know. But, oh, mother, can you imagine how I felt when father read that?"

Joe looks at me, and our eyes signal each other to let her have it.

"I don't know why the wounds are sweeter," gulps Peg, "but, oh, mother, oh, father, can you imagine how proud I felt when you read it?"

*   *   *   *   *

No way can I respond to anything Peg says these days without being responded to with tsk-tsks and exasperated sighs. If I think for a minute before I answer her in an effort to avoid her disdain, she tsk-tsks me double. "Being tired is a way of life for you, isn't it, mother?"

Sometimes it seems the only safe thing to do is not respond to her at all, but that only intensifies the hopeless shakings of her head and her angry stompings from the room.

I am about to tell Peg off when suddenly it dawns on me what has happened between us. I have been sacrificing everything to finish the book I am writing—Joey's book—toiling till midnight and then rolling out of bed in the morning and right on down the stairs to my typewriter. I talk to Peg absent-mindedly when she gets home from school and whirl back to my thesaurus. Instead of watching television with her at night, I scramble off to my study to finish one more chapter.

"It's just for a few weeks this fall, honey. You understand, don't you?"

She says she understands.

"Your patience can be your contribution to Joey's book, Peggie, your—"

Peg explodes. "I really understand what you're saying, mother, but it doesn't change the way I feel. I mean, suppose I said to you, 'I'm gonna be very busy the next few days. I'm sorry, but it's very important that I do so and so. So I'm not gonna have time to talk to you. I'm not gonna have time for you at all, but of course you know I love you.'

"You might understand, but how would you feel? You wanna know how I feel? How I feel is that you love me when I don't get in your way, which I do an awful lot of the time."

I remember with sadness how often Peg and I have gone to the mall together and she has wanted to stop to oooh and aah over a stationery sale or to watch the little children ride the train. And I have rushed her past these enticements, even in ordinary times, and she has said, "You're always in a hurry, aren't you, mother?" Once she said, "Just wait till I'm gone.

You won't have to bother with me any more. You won't have me around to bother you."

I remember, too, all the times she's been cleaning her room and been waylaid by a hundred alluring necessities. She starts to put away her Snoopy pad, but cannot do it till she dashes off a note to Jenny, her new best C.F. friend. She begins to dust her dresser, but first she must rearrange her earring tree, the teardrops on the first limb, the dots on the second, hers on one side, mine on the other. "Oh, mother, isn't it the most dazzling thing?"

I remember not speeding her along but sitting on her bed and asking how Jenny's lungs were doing. I remember the extra minutes I have taken endless times to walk from my room to hers to hang my loops on the third limb of the right side of her golden earring tree.

How much more sustaining the second memories are than the first. If I could live the last sixteen years over and do one thing differently, I would spend more time with Peggie. Nothing profound. Nothing difficult or costly. I would just spend more time really with Peggie.

* * * * *

Peggie smiles experimentally into the mirror in the dentist's office, and this stranger smiles back—a big, straight-toothed, Pepsodent-white smile.

Some people, it seems, have four-tooth smiles, and some people have six-tooth smiles, and some have eight-tooth smiles. Peggie, unfortunately, is an eight-tooth smiler. The capping of her teeth has been a long, painful process. But no matter; her old, gray, crooked teeth are no more.

I expect Peg to smile on and on at the other girl in the mirror, but she takes one hasty look, thanks the dentist, oh so politely, and clomps out the door.

Young people have to wait till they're sixteen to get their teeth capped. It takes all I clear on my first year's royalties on my first book to pay for Peg's caps, but I am thrilled that the only extra money Joe and I have in our marriage comes in her sixteenth year. All those years when the kids asked her, tittering, why she didn't brush her teeth are over, and right at Christmas time, too.

"I didn't see anything wrong with my teeth the way they were," Peg grumbles when we get to the car. "You were the only one who wanted me to get them capped."

At the same time he finished the capping, the dentist flicked out the last of Peggie's baby teeth. Sheepishly she puts it under her pillow. Once she lost a tooth when she was in the hospital. Neither Joe nor I visited her that day, but when she looked under her pillow the next morning, the tooth was gone, and in its place gleamed ten polished pennies. The tooth fairy always knows.

When she looks under her pillow this time, she finds a whole roll of pennies wrapped in red and green tinsel with a note that says:

I give you a hundred pennies
    as a thank you for a hundred times a hundred happy smiles
    and in honor of my last visit to you.
Unlike Peter Pan, all normal boys and girls do grow up.

                               Love,
                               The Tooth Fairy

P.S. I like your new teeth, but I do not want to see any of them under your pillow. T.F.

Peggie files the note away in her folder marked *11th grade*.

Six months later we are driving home from Jenny's high school graduation. "It sure is nice," Peg chirps, "not to have people make fun of me any more because I have black teeth. I sure am glad I got my teeth capped."

Six months later Peg has said the first decent thing about her new teeth—and in the process, of course, admitted to the indecency of the old.

"I mean, do you know how nice it is to be able to open your mouth and not be thinking that people are wonderin' what's wrong with your teeth—especially when you open your mouth as much as I do?"

*   *   *   *   *

Everybody was kidding me at school today, mother." Peggie is finally going to tell me the news that has been sprouting all over her face since she walked in the door.

"You remember how we had this value chart in mythology, mother?"

I remember all right. She has talked about nothing but the chart for days, carrying it around at school and making her friends compare the relative value they place on such items as God, family, humility, ingenuity, courage.

"Well, you know, there's this boy in mythology who arranged the items the exact same way I did? Richie? Well, he asked me today if I wanted to go to the Shakespeare Festival with him." Peg covers her face with her hands. "What will father say? He'll have a fit, won't he? He'll have an absolute fit."

I ask her why her father should be upset about her going out with such a nice boy.

"Well, you know how he is, so protective, and it being my first date and all. All the kids at school were telling me how to act, like I should be late getting ready and make Richie wait. But I do not intend to start a relationship playing games. And I told him no way could he sit at the curb and honk for me, that he had to come in and meet you guys.

"You know how Mary is always acting dumb? She acts dumb so much I think she almost believes it. Can that happen, that you become like what you act you are? But one day Mary's smartness is going to rebel, and then what will happen to her relationship with somebody who thinks she's dumb?

"Now I don't want you to get your hopes up, mother, even though he is tall and blond. And handsome, if you must know."

"Did I ever tell you tall or handsome was important?"

"No, and ya know I think it's better that you not start out being attracted to somebody physically, because you might not realize that's all you have. That's why I put youth and beauty at the bottom of my list of values. They don't last and then what?

"Guess what Judy said when I told her about Richie? She said, 'A senior, Peggie. Wow.' Like all that mattered was that he was a senior, not what kind of person he was. And all Denise could think about was that there was still time for him to ask me to the prom. Gladie just said, 'That's nice.' Good old Gladie.

"But what will father say? He'll die, won't he, mother? Father will just die."

When the night of Peg's first date arrives, father and mother both almost die of first-degree suspense. I don't go to bed at all, and Joe crashes downstairs the minute he hears Peg's hand on the doorknob. She's wearing her boots and her navy skirt and sky blue turtleneck and silver smiley-face earrings. With her hair blown and her face aglow with conquest, she shimmers in my moist eyes as the fairest of modern maidens.

"Well, I think I handled things well, if I do say so myself," she tells us. "Like when we got to the door. You know all the horror stories in the movies about what happens at the door. Well, Richie watches 'Star Trek,' too, so I put up my hand in the Vulcan hand salute and said, 'Peace. Live long and prosper.' Wasn't that a brilliant idea?"

Joe and I follow Peg's instructions on how to give the Vulcan hand salute. It isn't easy separating your fingers like that.

"There was just this one thing I didn't like. I mean, I think I'm a better driver than Richie, but he had to drive just because he's the guy. I don't suppose I could say, 'Next time it's my turn. We'll take my car, and I'll drive.' That wouldn't be good for his male ego, right?

"And I have to sit there all night and listen to him tell his boring stuff and act interested so I won't hurt his male ego? Doesn't anybody wonder about my ego? Can you imagine what years of this could do to a kid?

"I mean, he wasn't boring," she adds, blushing. "He was really nice and really smart, but what if he had been boring? I sat pretty far over on my side of the car so he wouldn't get any ideas.

"I enjoyed *Romeo and Juliet*. I think Richie had a good time, too, and I was glad of that. I suggested we exchange school pictures, and he got all excited."

On her picture Peggie writes, "Thanks for making my first date a memorable one. Don't ever change your value standards."

A week later Peg and Richie go to the Cleveland Natural History Museum—Peg, ego intact, waving jauntily as she perches on the green car cushion behind the wheel of our green car. She decides that Richie is awfully nice but that she does not want to get serious with him. "I think he's too smart for me, mother." He asks her to go to the prom, and she says no.

"The thing is, mother, that he likes me more than I like him. I can tell, because he lets things slip. You can't imagine the prestige of a junior going to the prom, but I don't think I should go because of the prestige, because he'd just think I liked him more. But I sure wish I could hang a sign on my back sayin' I was asked!"

* * * * *

P_{eg} comes with me to pick up my new typewriter. Her Memphis grandparents have given her some bonds, and she decides to use a portion of the interest from them to buy my old typewriter at its trade-in value. So we lug both typewriters home together, Peg immediately setting up office in her room and typing away with that nothing-but-ecstasy which is classic Peggie. How could she possibly have any misgivings that she might not adore every single thing about her typewriter? It's her first major purchase with her own money, isn't it? Well. . . .

```
This is the very first time that I have typed on my very own
typewriter! It cost me $105.00
type type type type type type type type type type type type
```

```
This is how one erases on this typewriter (with an erase
cartridge.) I am going to get a smiley face converter key!
```

Then she runs to give my typewriter a try.

```
Olympia, you give me the feeling that you are really well
made. I like you. Do you like me? Answer back. Yes ____
No ____ Are you going to be good and stay with us for a long
time?
```

```
Yes, as long as we all shall live.
```

```
Are backspaces traumatic for you?
```

```
They don't bother me now that I am young, but I understand
that older Olympians get a little shaken by frequent
backspacing.
```

```
How would you like a date with a Smith Corona?
```

```
Would I! When you sit in a warehouse all day, you don't
have much of a chance to develop relationships. I probably
should tell you, though, that when you took me home and
stopped in Sambos to eat, SC and I were in the back seat
together. We got quite well acquainted.
```

```
What do you think of Meg Woodson?
```

```
I'm familiar with her book IF I DIE AT THIRTY. I think
it's terrific.
```

```
Gotta stop now. Page line gauge tells me we are out of
room. Bye Bye.
```

Peg tells Joe she can make the type from her typewriter look like it came from an IBM. Joe tells Peg this is impossible. Peg slips her carbon cartridge into her machine and types:

```
I WAS WRONG!  I WAS WRONG!  I WAS WRONG!  I WAS WRONG!

       SIGNED BY  _____
```

She makes Joe sign his name and twirls about waving the paper over her head. "He was wrong!" she chants. "He was wrong! He was wrong! He was wrong!"

*   *   *   *   *

Peggie calls after school and asks me to pick her up. When I get there, Judy and Denise are with her, and she asks me to take them home, too. The three of them chatter away as we skid along the slick streets, but the minute we are alone, Peg clutches my arm.

"Oh, mother, I have this pain in my chest. It's a different kind of pain than I've ever had before. I got it in second period, and all day I didn't know whether I should call home or not, but I didn't want to miss English, and we were havin' a test in social studies."

"It's a pneumothorax," Dr. Rathburn diagnoses as soon as he looks at the x-ray. "A collapsed lung. What were you doing when you first felt the pain, Peggie?"

"I was goin' to sleep in chemistry."

"See what you get," chides Dr. Rathburn. He draws pictures for Peggie of exactly what has happened to her body and explains how they will attach her lung to her chest cavity so it cannot collapse again. When she leaves the hospital, her lungs should function on the same level as they did before.

Jenny is in the hospital too, lying in bed not moving and not talking, unable to keep anything in her stomach. "It's not like Patti," Peg assures me—and herself. "They think maybe they did something to Jenny's esophagus when they were fixin' her lung." Jenny is on her second pneumothorax.

"Peggie wants to room with Jenny. Should she be in there?" I ask the doctor.

"I think it would be good for Jenny to have Peggie in there."

The repair of a collapsed lung is routine. It is also painful. "Raise my bed," Peg whimpers. "Move my water closer. Lower my bed."

"Oh, Peggie, if I don't get some sleep, I'm going to be the next thing around here to collapse."

"If I'm such a burden to you, why don't you just go home?" Peg gestures wanly toward the door.

Taking care of Joey was never like this, I think. I only think it.

Kids with cystic fibrosis being friends with each other has

its disadvantages. They worry about each other. They worry about themselves when they see the disease advance in friends who are sicker than they. And how dreadfully are they damaged in spirit when C.F. friends die?

Still, Joe and I think the benefits outweigh the risks. "Can you imagine how good it is to be able to talk to someone about therapy and Dr. Rathburn and all?" Peg asks. "I mean, Jenny is my only good friend who understands if I say how bad carbenicillin smells."

I will always remember one C.F. mother who came to Joey's funeral. She was a casual friend, yet when she walked in, surrounded as I was by family and close friends, a kind of specialized wailing inside me was stilled.

As soon as Peg starts to feel better from her pneumothorax, she embarks on her getting-Jenny-to-eat mission. And, indeed, the day before Peg is dismissed, Jenny keeps down a big slice of pizza.

* * * * *

I read something today I think you'll like, Peg."

Adolescence is not the "silly age"; it is the splendid age, the age, when God, through the laws of nature puts in the young person's body and heart a deep call towards a body other than his own, towards a heart other than his own.

May every young person then have someone to explain this to him; parents who love him enough not to cling to him selfishly, but to direct his attention to the new and clear road along which "she" will appear.*

"Isn't that nice, honey?"

"It's okay."

"Just okay?"

"Well, you know. I feel funny talkin' about it."

"You mean because of the two bodies coming together?"

"Yeah. Do you think there's something wrong with me that I don't like boys the way other girls do? Do you think I need a psychologist?"

"Dr. Rathburn says some teenagers with C.F. get turned off to their own bodies because they're thin or not fully developed. They don't think they could ever turn anybody on, so as a protection they convince themselves they don't want anything to do with sex."

"Do you think glands have anything to do with it?"

"No. Do you?"

"No, but it's good to hear somebody else say so. Denise says she thinks the reason I don't think about boys all the time is because I have what I need at home, and also because I don't care what people think about me in that respect. She says a lot of sex stuff is forced on you because everybody expects you to do it.

"Ya know, there's this unmarried teacher in her late twenties at school, and she really likes being single, and she tells people she isn't married because she doesn't want to be married. Then people say to her, 'Well, don't you worry, honey. The right man will come along yet.' Can you imagine?

*Michael Quoist, *Prayers.* (New York: Sheed and Ward, 1965), p. 51.

"And you, mother. Don't think I don't know the only reason you want me to get married is so you can have grandchildren. You aren't thinking a bit about me, only about yourself."

"You're absolutely right, Peg. Please get married so I can have grandchildren."

"Every once in a while, mother, I get really tired of not being normal."

"You don't have to be like the majority of people in order to be normal, Peggie. Everybody doesn't have to have violent physical passions all the time because of some image that television or the kids hold in front of them. You have other passions. Be proud of what you are."

"Judy says John says I'm the most interesting person he knows. I'm glad he thinks that. Girls don't talk about anything but boys. Boys talk about girls, but they talk about other things, too."

Peggie has the word MAINTAIN cut out in big, blue letters fastened to the wall over her desk. "It's John's favorite word, mother. Sometimes when the kids come in my room they don't get it right away, but after a while they do. Actually, it's one of my favorite words too. It has a good sound—MAINTAIN."

Seventeen Years Old

Peggie says she doesn't want much for her birthday this year because, she says, she got too much for Christmas. She doesn't object, though, to our taking her to the Sveden House for dinner.

Joe and I know we cannot prepare Peg for the next world by making her mad for money and the things of this world that money can buy, but what if she doesn't have another birthday and we don't have another chance to buy her gifts?

"I don't think we ought to consider getting a colored TV," she lectures as we settle down at our table at the restaurant. "Like I enjoyed watching Lacey's colored TV in the hospital, but our not having one was what made it special. There ought to be one thing in your life you want that you don't have."

The light from the candle in our centerpiece flickers red and green and blue on her face, turning her into a television personality herself—a stern Miss Katherine shaking her finger at her "Romper Room" following. "You guys surprise me bein' such materialists," she scolds.

Actually, more than she is surprised by us, we guys are taken aback by her sudden disavowal of birthday presents and living color.

"Incidentally, mother," Peg goes on, "since that talk we had the other day on concessions, I decided I might get married if the right person came along."

I cannot remember any such talk. "What did I say about concessions, Peg?"

"About everybody having to make them. Nobody told me that before. I thought two people each did what they wanted and it came out right for them both, and I didn't see how I'd ever match with anybody that way. But if I gave up a little of myself for some guy, and some guy changed a little of what he was for me, we might fit."

I remember Peggie's comment of just a few months ago when the president made one of his energy conservation speeches. "I don't think he knows how hard a time he's gonna have. Doesn't he realize there's a whole generation of us out here who have never sacrificed anything?"

Peggie is growing up. At seventeen, is Peggie growing beyond us?

* * * * *

I didn't even get homesick for you guys," Peg whoops as we bring her home from her first looking-for-a-college trip. "Hardly," she whispers.

"Well, good. We didn't miss you either—much."

"What did you do with yourselves anyway?"

"Well, you might say your mother and I more or less went to bed early," Joe answers smugly.

"Honestly, father. I got enough sex at that college. Like the girl I roomed with had this huge button that said *Ya Wanna Pet?* Well, I could take that, but she had it next to a picture of Christ on the cross. Now that made me nervous.

"I mean, at chapel this guy with a guitar was teaching the kids a song he wrote about God and all, and he was nationally famous, but the kids were sitting there doing their homework. I just wanted to get out of there. What on earth are you going to do when I leave, mother?"

"Oh, I'm looking forward to doing a lot of things, like finally taking those courses in literature."

"Yeah, that's good. I'm glad you can do that."

Other things bother Peggie about the college she visited, like her roommate just grunting at her in the morning and Peg having to find the cafeteria by herself. "One time my roommate ate with me, and then when somebody asked me where I was from, she said, 'Oh, she's just a high school junior.' Like I was completely unimportant. Me and my friends outgrew that kind of lack of tact when we were in junior high.

"And all the kids dress like burnouts. I mean, not one person on that campus blow-dries their hair. Am I a snob? Beep. Beep-beep." The antenna has broken off Peg's portable radio, and she straddles the desk chair in her room with the silver rod fastened to the top of her head.

I tell Peg about how I stopped in a neighborhood church and knelt to pray the day she was gone. I cried a little, and a lovely young girl walked up from the back of the church and sat next to me for a minute. "I saw you were crying," she said, touching my arm, "and I just want to say I'm sorry for what's bothering you. But God loves you, so don't worry too much."

"That's the kind of girl I'd like you to go to college with, Peg."

"Yeah. I mean, she didn't say everything was going to be all right, and she was nice and polite. Not that I know that much stuff myself. I know *please* and *thank you* and that's about it. I don't want to go anywhere where they watch how you eat your soup."

We go down to the family room where Joe is reading, and the conversation turns to make-up. "I bet Peggie would look nice with a little make-up," Joe volunteers.

"I wear make-up, father!"

Joe gives her a careful once-over. "So you do, and it looks nice, honey."

"I'm not wearing it now," Peg shrieks, rolling on the floor till her antenna falls off. "Beep. Bee-ee—"

* * * * *

I go in to talk to Dr. Rathburn when he and Peg are done with their private visit. "Will Peggie make it through college?" I ask him, my heart dancing and dying as it dances and dies every time I press for a prognosis.

Dr. Rathburn answers, as he always answers, that he can prognosticate nothing. That some kids he is sure will not live through high school survive graduate school. And that he thinks Peg should go off to college if she only lasts six months.

"Peggie has one thing going for her that I can't overemphasize the importance of," he tells me, "and that's her pizazz. I have other patients whose lungs are in the same shape Peg's are in who are curled up in a ball someplace waiting to die. But Peggie comes in here and tells me how she's going to find the right college and major in English and be an editor at your publisher when she graduates."

An editor, eh? At my publisher?

"John found out about *If I Die*," Peg tells me as we stop in the hospital cafeteria for her usual doctor-visit snack of mashed potatoes and gravy. "I'm not wild to have my friends read it, because they get so shook in the first chapter when they find out how serious C.F. is. I sure don't want anybody feeling sorry for me.

"Like this teacher discovered I had C.F. the other day, and he came up to me after class and said, 'Have you been battling this affliction all your life?' It made me sick.

"People like that don't understand that I'm used to bein' the way I am. You know how June is deaf, and there's gonna be an operation soon that will make her hear, but she doesn't want the operation? Now me and June understand that, but nobody else understands.

"John says when he gets depressed, he reads my book. When he needs cheering up, he reads my book about death! Can you imagine? It's sad kids have to be sad. The counselor at school says the number one problem in high schools these days is depression.

"Ya know, I was wondering about that, and I decided one reason kids get depressed is that they feed their spirits junk food, like artificial preservatives and coloring that's unnatural. It doesn't belong in there. That's why I don't go to R movies. I haven't thought of that stuff yet, so why give myself night-mares? Once it gets into your head, you can't get it out, so why let it in?

"Did you know that absolutely all Denise thinks about is boys? Now I know it's normal to think about boys a lot, but with absolutely no time left for her to think about God, no wonder she's miserable."

I tell Peg that a part of people's depression is the helpless-ness and hopelessness they feel when it comes to being all they want to be. "I'm trying to write a book, Peg, about one human spirit that's climbing high—and a young, overloaded human spirit at that."

"My book? My second book? That sounds pretty good—why you're writing it, I mean. Oh, boy, a book to make people happy.

"Ya know, all this time I thought my health would be getting worse, but I'm getting better instead. Do you think me bein' happy has anything to do with that?"

*   *   *   *   *

How's Lacey?" Peggie asks one of the secretaries from the C.F. office.

"Lacey died, Peggie."

"I thought so," says Peg.

"I'm going to write a note to Lacey's mother," she tells me. Her first sympathy note. "What did people write to you when Joey died that helped the most?"

I tell her that one of the things that helped was people saying they missed Joey, too.

Peg hunches over her daisy stationery for twenty minutes before she brings her note to me for approval.

Dear Mrs. Smith,

I heard that Lacey died. I'm sorry. I know you miss her, but I know she is happy in heaven, and I'm sure my brother gave her a big welcome.

I will miss Lacey too, especially when I'm in the hospital or when I watch a John Denver special on colored T.V.

Love,
Peggie

"Whew!" sighs Peg. "That's a lot harder to do than you might think."

A few weeks later I watch her painstakingly gift-wrap a set of Snoopy postcards. "Whose birthday, Peg?"

"Well, it would have been Patti's in a few days. I've been sending Patti's mother a present on Patti's birthday for two years now. I mean, I know how you guys feel on Joey's birthday. Wouldn't it help you if someone sent you a present?"

But you're helping yourself, too, aren't you, Peg? You always sent Patti a present on her birthday, and in your own way you're sending her one again.

Patti's mother remembers Peggie's birthday, too. And Christmas and Easter. Is she, too, sending presents to Patti?

* * * * *

I come home from speaking at my publisher's sales conference, and Joe and Peg meet my plane, waving and grinning as though I am their personal celebrity.

"Wait till you hear the exciting thing that happened," I gush. "In my introductory remarks I told the people about what Dr. Rathburn said about the importance of pizazz, and how you intend to become an editor for them when you finish college, Peg. And all these executives came up to me afterward and said, 'Tell Peggie we'll be looking for her five years from now.'"

"Did they really mean it?" gasps Peg. "Or were they just saying it 'cause I'm a kid—like being nice? Oh, wouldn't that be wonderful?" Peg clasps her hands to her meager bosom and comes to an awed halt in the middle of the horde of travelers surging toward baggage claim at Cleveland Hopkins Airport.

I will never forget the kindness of these people to my daughter. Did they sense how important it is to a young girl without much time to live to have that time all planned out?

Later in the afternoon I hear Peg talking to one of the neighborhood girls who does therapy on her. "Isn't that great, having it all settled? They start bugging you about careers in the fourth grade. I mean, they say you don't have to decide then, but they sure keep bugging you. Boy, I can plot my whole college course now."

As the day wears on, Peg voices a few reservations. "Ya know, I've been thinking about this job, mother. How much do they pay? Could I have an apartment like Mary Tyler Moore if I worked there? And how about being bored? I wouldn't want to start at the bottom. And do they have women in power?"

Still, from this day she sets the sails of her heart toward a certain, coveted landfall.

* * * * *

Often Peggie and I have our most meaningful conversations in Teddi's restaurant as she devours a hot roast beef sandwich. Well, we are in Teddi's, and Peg is devouring her regular, and I am conversing with her about Christ's parable of the sheep and goats. Of how He said He'd judge us to be sheep or goats on the basis of our treatment of the sick and the homeless and the hungry.

If I communicate anything to Peggie before she ventures out into our success-oriented society, it ought to be what success is before God. "What do you think this parable has to do with the career goals of the kids at school, Peggie?"

But Peggie does not converse back. "How should I know?" she shrugs.

"Well, you might give it a little thought."

"I thought. I still don't know."

"Boy, Peg. You get all enthusiastic about my writing another book about you, but you surely don't cooperate when I try to talk to you about something."

"Well, you ask such dumb questions. When I was thirteen, all this stuff about God was new to me. You're gonna have to think up questions that aren't so dumb."

She calls me dumb once too often. "Well, maybe we better forget the book altogether."

"Well, maybe we better." Peggie consumes the rest of her roast beef sandwich in silence, eyes burning bright, occasionally lifting from her prey to glitter through me, keeping me out of the cave of safety to which my spiritual hounding has driven her.

I've talked to Peg before about the least of Christ's brothers. First I mentioned my friend Susan and how she befriended the lost souls of the earth. "She doesn't know they're lost souls, though, Peg."

"I think that's the only way it can work."

Then a week or so ago I read her C. S. Lewis's response to a comment on a boring friend. "Yes, but let's not forget that our Lord might well have said, 'As ye have done it unto one of the least of these my bores, ye have done it unto me.'"

SEVENTEEN YEARS OLD   *139*

Peggie said nothing.

A pattern emerges. Me, new thought; her, sensitive reaction. Me, same thought; her, no reaction. Me, same thought again; her, hostile reaction.

I eye Peg obliquely to see if she is emerging from her lair, and her eyes meet mine with a frolicsome symmetry. "It's all right if you repeat yourself, mother. After all, you're in your forty-seventh year. You're bound to forget things in your *forty-seventh* year."

* * * * *

The kids at Patterson Christian are really nice," Peg tells us, leaning over into the front seat of the car as we bring her home from her second looking-for-a-college excursion. "I mean, they didn't have red hearts painted on their mattresses saying *Sex with Bob*, and they had Betsey Clark pictures up and quotations and things.

"I don't know when I had so much fun. Like here it is the end of May, and last night we all went out for ice cream with winter hats on.

"I don't think I'll have any special friends at Patterson right away, though. I didn't come across anybody who likes to talk deep. But the kids will be nice to me."

We pull off the highway and into a Holiday Inn for supper. In the restaurant, Peg plunks an elbow on the table, plunges her head into her hand, and says, "What have you guys been thinkin' while I've been gone?" A Rodin statue talking.

"Profanity isn't allowed, father. But ya know, you can say everything you want to say without profanity. Some of it sounded funny, though. Like they kept saying, 'Boy, that ticked me off.' I don't suppose you guys know what they say at Sub West instead of *ticked* off?

"No? I didn't think so. Tsk-tsk. Dumb, dumb, dumb."

"I understand," Joe says, "that the time eventually comes when they start thinking their parents know something again."

"Oh, I wouldn't really say you guys are dumb. Just that your knowledge is a bit outdated."

If this is what forty-eight hours at college do to her, how will we survive four years?

Then Peg leans across the table and lowers her voice. "There was one interesting thing I learned in this philosophy class I went to, father. I mean, did you know you can't tell there's not an elephant in this room?"

Joe's eyes probe the dusky depths of the restaurant. "I can't know there's not an elephant in this room?"

"Well, father, if I had my notebook with me, I could prove to you that you can't know there's not an elephant in this room."

While Joe pays the bill, Peg draws me into the souvenir shop. "Let's look at the toyth, mommy," she lisps. And then, "The only thing I'm gonna have to get used to is walkin' around in my underwear."

"You know, honey, your arms do not look skinny at all any more."

"They don't? Ya mean it?" She hurtles into the ladies' room and almost into the mirror. "Hey, they don't, do they? I mean, maybe with a sleeveless top they might a little, but they really look normal with this top. For the first time I have slender arms, not skinny.

"Hey, world, Peggie Woodson's arms are regular!"

"Incidentally, Peg," I tell her when we get back in the car, "I thought of what the kids at high school say instead of *ticked* off."

"What does it begin with?"

"P."

"Very good, mother. Very contemporary."

* * * * *

A letter arrives saying that New York grandmother and grandfather have sold their home on Long Island and are moving to Florida.

"But the hedges! Who will trim the hedges?" Peg cries. "And will they still be *New York* grandparents or what?"

We have spent almost every summer vacation since Peg was born on Long Island. She has lived in three houses in her seventeen years, but it is against the maple tree in the back yard of the little house surrounded by hedges that she has measured her growth.

"Why are the hedges so important to you, Peg?"

"Well, you know how every year we all see who can spot the house first, and I'm always the one, and I spot it from way off because of the tall hedges."

"Maybe it's because the hedges enclose the house and seem to stand for a place of safety and love."

"Well, if you were analyzing something like this in a book, that is the sort of thing you'd say."

"Look at that lady with the shopping bag," Peg is wont to squeal in the mall. "She's wearin' a top just like New York grandmother wears. Doesn't she look just like a grandma?"

"Why do you like older folks so much, Peg?"

"Because they're nice to you, and they don't care if you're funny lookin'."

I suggest to Peg that while we will always miss the house on Long Island, it's grandmother and grandfather who give us a sense of permanency, and that in time any house they live in will grow hedges around it in our hearts.

"What mush!" snorts Peg, but gradually she feels better about Florida. "Can't you see those two cute things riding their three-wheel bikes under the palm trees?"

Joe talks on occasion about finding another church.

"I'm not movin'," Peg spouts. "If you guys move, I'm getting an apartment in Cleveland. The thing is, though, I don't have money for an apartment. But I'm still not movin'. I'd never have a room of my own again. I mean, I'd have a room with my stuff in it, but it wouldn't be my room."

Peg and I sit at the kitchen table making fish for her Sunday school class out of paper plates and elbow macaroni and talking about a cousin who is getting married. He has drifted in and out of job after job, and we worry that he'll meander in and out of marriage in the same way. I tell Peg that I think our cousin's problem is that nothing he does is lifted out of the ordinary.

Peg wants to know how you give something a meaning beyond the thing itself, and I tell her it's by doing it for the glory of God.

"I bet none of my friends ever thought of that," yells Peg. "How come you never talked to me about that before?"

I never talked to you about *that* before, Peggie? Remember when you got all excited about clapping for God? "Well, maybe I did, honey, and you weren't ready to hear it the way you're ready now."

"Boy, I'd much rather get good grades in math for God than good grades for me." Peggie is taking an algebra course at the community college this summer. "Oh, mother, I wonder if there's other good stuff you assume I know just because you know it. What could it be?"

The sun, which rarely shines in Cleveland, blazes through the red and blue curtains on the kitchen window and onto Peg's upturned face. I think of William Wordsworth's lines:

> My heart leaps up when I behold
> A rainbow in the sky.

I tell Peg there's a verse in the Bible that says that whether we eat or drink or whatever we do, we should do it all to the glory of God, and Peg gives me nine-and-a-half minutes till "All My Children" comes on to find where the verse is located.

"Remember how Tara was married to Philip, then Chuck, then Philip again, mother? Well, Donna, who married Chuck after Tara, and Philip are both afraid Tara's getting interested in Chuck again. And David poisoned his wife, who he thought he divorced but didn't, and Nick took off for Chicago after he told Erica he would marry her because she was dying, and

. . . I'll tell you one thing—characters in soap operas sure don't do things for God's glory."

"Okay, Peg, go watch your soap opera, but clean up this macaroni gloop first."

"Now put that in, mother. If you're gonna write up this conversation for our book, put in that you couldn't keep from saying that. Why can't I clean up the table during a commercial?"

"You know, Peggie, this morning I asked God to show me once and for all if we really were supposed to write another book. I suggested that if we were, maybe you and I could have a significant conversation today."

"Oh, come on. Get out of here. God never gives me signs. Do you know how long it's been since we had a significant conversation?"

The next morning at dawning Peg soars into my room. "Ya know how for two days I've been working on that one stupid math problem, mother, and it would not come out right? I mean, I must have done that problem a thousand times, and I asked Judy how, and I asked Denise how, and I just couldn't get it. Well, when I got up a while ago, I said a little prayer about it, and it came out right the very next time—and right after we were talking about doing stuff for God. You're not impressed, are you, mother?"

"I'm impressed. I'm impressed."

"I mean, that's not the kind of thing I do. That's the kind of dumb thing you do. And it came out perfect the very next time." Peg perches on the hamper in the hall as she gets dressed, an early-morning songbird fluting and fluttering with the excitement of a new day.

As Peg matures, I wait for her to lose the wonder with which she's always greeted spiritual discovery. Today I dare hope that rupture will never occur.

Peg goes into reverie. "You know what I think it is to glorify God? I think it's like you're sitting in school, and there's somebody you like or admire a lot, maybe just a friend or maybe a boyfriend or a teacher, and you keep saying nice things about them. If anybody mocks them out, you tell them to shut up or explain why they're wrong, and whenever that person's name is mentioned, you build them up. Now transfer all that to God, and that's glorifyin' Him.

"Now don't go getting sick about this, mother, like making a speech or something. Sometimes when you talk about God you get this tone in your voice like you're lookin' at a newborn baby, and that is another of your tones I cannot stand."

"Guess what, mother?" she chirps later when she flies in from the community college. "You'll never guess what Maxi the genius said when I asked her how you could do your math for God's glory? I mean, we were rushing down the hall, and I asked her out of the blue, and she says, 'Well, let's say a man builds a race car, and it's the fastest race car ever built. Vroom!' I couldn't believe dignified Maxi going vroom vroom!

"And then she says, 'This race car is the best. Everyone praises the builder for creating such a fantastic car. Well, it's the same way with a person. If someone is a terrific person, people should praise God because God made him.'

"It would take Maxi to think up something like that, right, *ma?* I mean, I just want to be the best possible Peggie Woodson, so let's not get all mushy about it, *ma.*"

I look up the rest of the rainbow poem.

> My heart leaps up when I behold
>   A rainbow in the sky;
> So was it when my life began;
> So is it now I am a man;
> So be it when I shall grow old,
>   Or let me die!
> The Child is father of the Man;
> And I could wish my days to be
> Bound each to each by natural piety.

* * * * *

What nice things do you really think about me, mother?" Peg flops on the bed beside me, all loose joints and jeans worn limp, but with a hard-souled longing in her voice.

"Well, I think you have high moral standards and deep spiritual sensitivity."

"Beam, beam," beams Peg.

"And you choose nice friends, and you're happy and sad with them. And you have an inquiring mind and an outstanding academic record."

"Hey, this is pretty good. Have we done this sort of thing before, mother?"

"And you're responsible in your driving and on your job."

"More, more."

"Well, let's see. You're just a fine young girl, and I'm proud when I see you becoming a fine young woman."

"Running down, huh?"

"How about that you're pretty? Though that's not terribly important."

"You never told me that before," Peg breathes, sinks her face in my pillow, and sobs.

"I must have told you that, honey. You were a darling baby and the cutest little girl. I've always thought you were pretty."

"I don't know what's the matter with me. I don't know why I'm acting like this."

An interesting coincidence: Joe took me to a play last night. I'd worked hard at looking nice, and Joe said, "My goodness, Meg, you're beautiful." He'd never said that to me before. I walked and talked all night as though I were beautiful all the way through. The play we saw? *My Fair Lady*.

Well, some of us embodied spirits may put spiritual fairness at the top of our value charts, but we still value fairness of body.

"You do think my senior pictures will turn out good, don't you, mother?" Peg's tears turn into an entreaty that lifts her out of my pillow and sits her upright. "Come on, I have to hear it. They'll come out nice, won't they?"

How could her senior pictures miss? What with the blouse

purchased for the occasion, the blue a perfect match to her azure eyes. We even bought new pants, though they wouldn't show in the picture. Even new glasses with pink and blue shell frames, wire frames being out now. Fortunately, it was time for a trip to the eye doctor anyway.

"I got my senior picture taken for the glory of me, didn't I, mother? But then I'm only seventeen. I'll improve with time."

"Too bad the picture won't show your legs, Peg. You have exceptionally good legs."

"So what you're telling me is that my senior pictures will come out good? Like on a scale of one to ten, how good? Mmm, good legs, you say, so skinny and all? Boy, I really appreciate your telling me that, mother."

* * * * *

Aunt Lynn again flies us to California for a visit. While we're there, a niece has us over for hamburgers, and after supper Peg wanders outside to explore.

Suddenly she streaks back in. "Oh, mother, there's a hawk in the field outside—a real hawk. He stands on this man's finger, and then he flies around the field and comes back and lands on the man's finger again. You gotta see this, mother."

I am helping my niece clear the table, and I do not follow Peggie.

Later in the back seat of the car she carries on and on about the hawk.

"That was really important to you, wasn't it, Peg?"

"Well, it was just like in books. Haven't you read about trained hawks in books?"

"I'm sorry I didn't come look."

"I never saw a hawk before." Peg's voice quivers. "It's just that you never get excited about anything, mother."

We go to the circus, and I try to atone for the hawk by gasping in horror as a trapeze artist fumbles on the high wire.

"He did it on purpose," scoffs Peg, disgusted by my naïveté. She lets me buy her a pennant pencil at the souvenir stand, but we both know she is patronizing me.

At midnight we stand on Aunt Lynn's patio, the lights of the San Gabriel Valley glistening below. "I think circuses are mostly for little kids," Peg tells me. "I mean, I kept wondering if the clowns and all were really happy, and little kids don't do that."

"Isn't this view fantastic, Peg?"

"It's okay. It's pretty the way a Christmas tree is pretty. I'd rather look at a plain tree."

A sense of sadness and loss as old as the first mother settles around me like the night. Oh, Peggie, you've left most of the magic of childhood behind you. There won't be many more times you'll dash back from an adventure and holler for me to come and see. And there will never be another time for me to run with you to an open field to watch a hawk circle to its master and to dream with you of all the faraway booklands in which you have traveled and in which hawks have circled.

Peggie drives to the doctor by herself—first time —and comes home noisy with importance. "Guess how much I weighed," she bellows. "You'll never guess. Just guess."

"Ninety-three?" Ninety-three being her all-time high, but one she lost a while ago in the normal ups-and-downs of C.F.

"Guess again."

"It can't be ninety-five."

"It is! Ninety-five! You know how Dr. Rathburn always writes down what I say? Well, I made him write that down in my folder, so he put down *95—new record*, and I got out my red pen and starred and circled it.

"He said I had stuff in my lungs, and I said, 'Where?' And he said, 'All over,' and I said, 'Tough. I'm feeling good, eating great, and gaining weight, so tough.' And he said physical examinations were not always conclusive."

"Was he in a good mood?"

"Well, maybe not when I got there, but when I left, yes. He came out to the waiting room and asked where you were. I just said I came by myself. I wasn't gonna make a big thing out of it.

"I might as well tell you, mother," she goes on, no quieting of her voice indicating a shift in her own good mood, "that everybody I know with C.F. died since the last time I was over there."

This has become a routine report. Exaggerated, of course. And, of course, never routine.

"Oh, honey, who?"

"Well, cute little Bonnie who wrote the poem on the hospital napkin for one. And Josh Holt, the older guy who was always riding Joey piggyback in the hospital. Now don't go gettin' all soupy on me, mother.

"Is father at the church? I want to tell you two guys something together. Why don't you get on the upstairs phone and I'll call him up?

"Guess what, you guys. My pulmonary function score is 69."

"That's wonderful, Peg," says Joe. I am unable to say anything. Peg's vital capacity has been in the lower fifties for years.

Peg comes looking for me and puts her arms around me, patting my shoulder with quick, butterfly-light taps. "For goodness sakes, mother, you're not gonna lose me right away, ya know."

"Sometimes I worry about why you don't cry more when your friends die, Peg."

"I cry. But if you want me to be depressed for a month every time someone with cystic fibrosis dies, I'll be depressed all my life. You know how they say that sometimes C.F. patients die in clumps? Well, I bet we've had our clump for a while. I bet no more of us kids with C.F. die for a long time now.

"You really ought to try being optimistic for a change, mother. I tell ya, being optimistic is a lot more fun than being pessimistic."

Joe comes galloping home to hear Peg's good medical report in person, but she moves on to other things, digging in her purse and coming up with her program for the new school year. "Look at this, father. All the stuff I wanted fit— advanced English and French and arts seminar and Shakespeare and science fiction and speedwriting. I can't believe it.

"Do you think God had anything to do with all these good things that have been happening? Oh, I'm sure He did, this being the beginning of my senior year and all."

* * * * *

Peggie's advanced English class prepares to spend four days at Mohican State Park, communing with nature, writing poetry, and such things. Peg is wild to go until she learns that you can't choose who your cabin mates will be, and then she wails, "No way am I goin'. No way am I gonna let those kids see me get therapy and all. I mean, the nicest kids in the senior class are in advanced English, but a lot of them in there are creeps, too."

But soon Peg changes her mind again. "I'm goin' anyway! I'll ask the teacher to let me have Gladie in with me to do therapy. I'll tell him I need Denise, too, which is mostly true, because Glad has never done therapy before and her arms probably wouldn't hold up.

"That'll only leave one person in my cabin I can't control. I'm goin'! There's nobody in that class I can't live with for four days if I have to, right, mother?"

How I wish the best for Peg as she *goes to meet the foe,* and in the light of past woundings, how I worry about the worst that could happen, a regular fellow-feeler myself. Only more than that—a mother feeling for her daughter, a feeling no dictionary has a term for.

Peg's peer-panic, as I've come to think of it, goes back to her kindergarten days, when she first safaried into the public domain. There were not many children her age on our block, but a few houses down from us between our house and the school was a house full of children of all ages. What an inviting racket they made as they tumbled together in their front yard, but whenever Peg walked by they yelled, "Here she comes. Run! Run!" And they jumped up and ran to their back yard.

Peggie, being Peggie, ran after them. "Why won't you play with me?" she shouted.

"We don't like the stuff in your mouth," they shouted back, pressed against the safety of their patio wall. "Our mother told us not to. Peggie, go home!" Time after time, "Here she comes. Run! Run!" Nor did Joe's talking to the children's parents accomplish a thing.

Sometimes I think Peg's tender five-year-old heart was violated in a way that does not allow for full repair. And then through the years the Eugenes and their kin sprayed their venom and their avoidance in the raw places.

I pray in the days preceding Mohican that God will control who Peg's fourth cabin mate will be, and I pray in the days during Mohican that God will help Peg see the good in the kids she looks down on—so sure they will reject her that she must reject them first.

"You know the fourth girl in my cabin, mother?" Peg asks on the day following Mohican. "Well, it was like a miracle, almost like meeting another one of me. I mean, I'm fifth in class rank and Betty's fourth. I have C.F., and Betty has chronic bronchitis and coughs all the time, and she thinks there's something else you can do in life if you don't want to get married, too.

"In school I thought Betty was one of the tough kids, but when we were up on this hill and I was freezing, she stood behind me to shelter me from the wind. And when I got a ride down the hill, she ran all the way down because she realized she had the key to the cabin and I wouldn't be able to get in."

Of course I have to tell Peg Who was responsible for assigning Betty to her cabin. Once again she will be gratefully impressed with how mother's prayers get through.

But Peg throws mother's prayers back in mother's face. "I really think that what happened would have happened whether or not you prayed, and I must say I wish you would stop trying to control my life in this manner. You make me feel like I don't do anything myself.

"All the kids were so different from what I thought they were like, mother. I mean, there was this one kid I could not believe. At school he's a real troublemaker, but at Mohican he spent his time playing with the little kids from the next camp who were slow learners. And he baked cupcakes! Of which I ate my share!

"Everybody was so nice. I just got along with everybody. It will be interesting to see what they're like at school tomorrow. Actin' like their old selves I bet. But ya know, I'm not the only one who's afraid of getting made fun of. Like this one girl told me she spent two years learning to control her facial muscles so no one would know what she was feeling and mock her out."

Peg says she discovered that most of the kids do stuff like that. That the only way you can tell what they're thinking is from their eyes, and if they wear mirror glasses, you can't even tell then.

Only one bad thing happened while Peg was gone—she collapsed halfway up the Mohican mountain. "If I'd been swimming, I'd have drowned on the spot, mother. I sank to the ground, and I mean, I could not breathe. Can you imagine what it feels like when everybody else is on their way up a mountain and you're slidin' down?

"The last day I spent an hour sitting in a drizzle by the creek. I wrote a couple poems, if you'd like to see them."

Baren Branches

Gnarled branches reach
Out, trying in frustration
To snatch back their leaves.

Riverbank Weeds

Thirsting fronds reach for the
Water—
Searching for life.

I say nothing to Peggie about sitting in the rain. And I will say nothing to her about my continuing prayers that she will see the good in all the kids at school. At this point I do not need to enhance Peggie's confidence in God or mother—only Peggie's confidence in Peggie.

* * * * *

Did I ever tell you how Pete at youth group said that his idea of being filled with the Holy Spirit was that it was like a mood? You know how a mood colors your whole life—like anger? And when you're filled with the Holy Spirit, that's like a Holy Spirit mood. Well, I thought that sounded pretty good, and that's just what the festival was like.

"All the groups that sang had this certain air about them. I can't tell you how it felt. They kept smiling at each other, and you could tell they loved each other. I'd say it was a peace, but everybody says that so often, it doesn't mean much.

"Do you ever go out in the back yard by yourself with the trees all around and listen to the birds, mother? Well, the Holy Spirit mood was something like that.

"And the kids had it, too. I mean, there were three thousand people there, and everybody you'd talk to would love you even if they didn't know you. I never got hugged so much in my life, and all those kids singing together, 'Ain't it grand to be a Christian?'

"Can't you drive this car any faster, mother? I know father will want to hear all this." The Jesus Jubilee tops Mohican as the trip of the year.

"Well, after a while I left Pat and went out to get a doughnut," Peg goes on, referring to the girl from Patterson College who had invited her back to the school for the concert. "But when I came back in, I couldn't find my seat, so I just happened to sit in this other place. And we were holding hands, and we were singing this song, 'I want to love you, Jesus,' and my row was the only row that put their hands up when we sang that.

"Now you know me, I'm getting to be a non-emotional person, but when we did that, I started to cry, and I could not stop. That was the Holy Spirit comin' into me, wasn't it, mother? The presence of God you're always talking about? For a while I wasn't sure if it was just emotion, but it wasn't like anything I experienced before. I mean, it was like strength and joy coming into me from the guy next to me."

Neither Peg nor I notices that we have missed our exit on the interstate till the skyscrapers of downtown Cleveland cast their unjolly-gray-giant shadows over us. It takes us an extra hour to get home, but nothing shadows Peggie's sunny skies.

"You know why I think that sort of thing hasn't happened to me too much, mother? Because I wouldn't let it. I was afraid something weird would go on, and I don't like to lose control. Also, you know how Ken Medema sings, 'Why Am I Afraid to Love'? What if I asked and didn't get it?

"Most of the jokes they told were about preachers. I mean, this one guy imitated a minister at the beginning of a Sunday service. 'We are gathered here to worship' and all that, and he said it completely deadpan. And then he said, 'Isn't that exciting?' And everybody cracked up.

"But at that concert I got sung at and preached at for twelve hours, and I didn't get bored. We were heathens this morning. We didn't go to church. No sense in killing it."

As the weeks following the concert pass, the house spins with its music, figuratively and literally as Peg sings and sways to the records and tapes she brought back with her.

> God gave rock and roll to you
> rock and roll to you

"Maybe He gave that beat to you, Peg, but not to me."

> Put it in the soul of everyone
> in the soul of everyone

"If I ascend up into the attic, it is there," quips Joe. "If I make my bed in the basement, behold, it is there."

"Ya know, mother, now that the Holy Spirit smacked me in the face the way He did at the music festival, I realize I've been feeling the presence of God all along, like at the early guitar service daddy's been having and whenever he gives the benediction. I just didn't recognize it.

"It doesn't last too long, though—never till the next Sunday. It's hard always to be aware of the presence. Like sometimes it leaves you slowly, and you don't know it's been gone till you get it back again."

Peg jumps up and puts a Larry Norman album on the stereo. "I was kind of surprised you were happy about what happened to me at the concert, mother," she screeches over the cacophony. "Knowing how you like dignity and liturgy and all."

"Well, honey, I'm just glad that what happened to you happened. A lot of kids have a hard time finding the reality of Christ in the particular form of Christianity in which they grew up. They say the words so often before it's possible for the words to have any meaning for them that it's hard for the words ever to have meaning for them. Of course, not all mothers would be as broad-minded as I." I yell the last sentence extra loudly.

"Nor as humble, mother! Can you hear me? Did you know I've started readin' the Bible a chapter a day every single day? Did you hear what I just said? This is Woodson talking here."

* * * * *

Peg uses the air compressor on which her aerosols work to blow up balloons for John's birthday, two large plastic bags of them. She goes to school early, and having secretly ascertained the combination of John's locker, stuffs it full of balloons. Then she stands in a corner and watches.

John opens his locker, and balloons shoot out like firecrackers, lighting on his head, on his books. John is on his hands and knees laughing and trying hopelessly to capture the bouncing bubbles of color. All the kids are screaming and jumping for balloons.

"Now that's the way a senior year should be," boasts Peg. "Everybody always says your senior year is your happiest, but my junior year was my happiest. I wish I had known so I could have enjoyed enjoying it more.

"You know what Lester says? He says that when you're a senior, it's always in the back of your mind that the end is coming, and he's right. Your senior year goes by so fast, and all the time you're thinkin' about graduation and knowin' that things are never gonna be the same again.

"And that's the pain of it," she adds solemnly. "Knowin' that things are never gonna be the same."

* * * * *

Valentine's Day is also Carnation Day at Suburban West. One of the service clubs sells the kids carnations, which are delivered anonymously to the recipients in their homerooms. Gladie is in charge of this year's project, and the proceeds go to cystic fibrosis. Peg receives five carnations.

"Almost more than anybody in the school, mother. I mean, my whole homeroom together only got ten. Everybody was lookin' at me in amazement. It's not wrong to be proud and feel this good, is it? No telling how long this will boost my morale."

I take a picture of Peg holding the five carnations under her chin, their blush highlighting the bloom of happiness on her cheeks.

"You know how the mothers at church are always worrying about whether their kids will follow their standards or go on drugs and stuff when they get in high school? Well, I don't think those mothers understand that a time comes when, if you have to choose between your peers and your parents, you stop and think. I've never figured out why friends are so important, but they are."

You're wobbling over the border of your own world, Peg. You know you have my love, but how lonely will you be out there on your own? Will you be judged as witty and wise and desirable as you need to believe you will be?

Peg sits on the hall steps with tears in her eyes because she doesn't want to go away from her friends. I remind her that she'll make new friends in college, but she doesn't see the point to that, because in four years she'll have to leave them, too. If she stays home, her friends will go away, and those who stay home will go to different schools, and the boys will get married, and even though she's just friends with them, things will be different.

"You know Nan, mother, who used to call me *my fiend Peggie* and *enemy Peggie?* Well, we're friends now, and I gave her this valentine on a string, and she sat all through lunch with the valentine hanging from one ear, eating a carnation. I don't know how I can leave friends like that."

Peg pauses and looks at me warningly. "Not you, mother. Just my friends."

"A part of your friends are a part of you, Peg. You can't leave them totally behind. Would you rather have no friends to leave?"

*   *   *   *   *

Hi, Peg. How was work?" I get home from my writers' workshop shortly after Peggie gets home from her insurance office.

"Questions, questions! That's all anybody does around here—ask questions!"

"Well, for goodness sakes, Peggie, I was just interested in how your day went."

"Ya know how you're still talking about that time I didn't call you for three weeks when I was in the hospital? You wanna know why I didn't call? I'll tell you why I didn't call. Because I knew what you'd say if I did. 'Are you getting enough to eat? What did you have for breakfast? What did you have for dinner? How was your pulmonary function test? What time did you get to bed? How much are you coughing?'

"I didn't want anybody checkin' up on me. Can you imagine what a good time I had for three weeks with nobody checking up on me?"

Well, I wouldn't have been checking up on Peg exactly. I certainly wasn't checking up on her now when I asked how her day went. Any question an adult asks Peg these days comes through to her as some kind of test.

Still, I think about what Peg is trying to tell me. I wouldn't consider reading her mail or rearranging her room or joining her parties, but do I pry and poke myself into her affairs in more subtle ways?

I do ask a lot of questions. "I see you got a letter from Jenny today. Did she have anything interesting to say? Who was that on the phone just now? Nothing going on between you and John I should know about, is there? Where did you and Denise go last night? Did you have a good time? When did you get in?"

"You're home a little later from your writers' workshop this afternoon than you usually are, aren't you, mother?" Peg asks cutely, not finished making her point with me. "What happened? Was Harold there? Did he read his science fiction? How was it?"

Peg doubles over laughing, incapacitated by her own ingenuity. "How about the psychiatrist—was she there? Did you have refreshments? Were they good? How much did you eat? When do you meet. . . ."

* * * * *

It's terrible the way they're cracking down on discipline at school this year, mother. Like if you're in the cafeteria and you want to go to the practice rooms, some guard will treat you like a criminal. 'Hey you, kid, where do you think you're going?'"

Joe and I regret the lack of senior privileges at the high school, convinced that the best thing teachers or parents can do for kids their last year at home is to remove external discipline and encourage them in self-discipline. Give them a trial run for all the years to come.

It's a hard thing for Joe and me to do, though, where Peggie's health is concerned. Peggie knew back in October that her flu shot was due, and crucial, but she purposely didn't tell us it was time to go to the doctor because she doesn't like shots.

Yet all the material we read on young adults with C.F. says that once parents let them be truly responsible for their own welfare, they are truly responsible. "Okay, Peggie," Joe concedes. "From now on you tell us when you want therapy. You decide if you're going to take your aerosols and your medications." We hold our breath to see if Peggie will hold on to her breath of life.

Of course, we can't relax with a single mandate the grip of terror with which we've held Peg for seventeen years. "Do you know what father said to me this morning in the bathroom?" Peg sputters. "He said should I be walking around in my bare feet, and didn't I want to put something on my cold feet? I mean, he asked me, but he was so tense it was like an order."

"Remember when daddy was doing therapy on you yesterday and you coughed up that blood, honey? I think that scared him. And when you were saying that your toenails were blue and that they'd never been blue before. Your father worries because he loves you."

"Yeah, well, they're my toenails. Don't you think I worry? And they're my feet after all. I oughta know if they're cold.

"Ya know, I was talking to this girl in a wheelchair at school the other day, and she was saying that kids with a handicap have a greater than ordinary need to be independent. And I said, 'Yeah, and the parents of kids with something wrong with them have a greater than ordinary need to keep them dependent.'"

But suddenly the flu season is upon us, and half Peg's school is out with a virus. "If I got this virus, it could be really bad, couldn't it?" Peg asks with a new big-scare in her voice.

"I was goin' to see this play at school tonight, mother—*The Drunkard*—but do you think I should stay home and go to bed early instead? I mean, me and my friends were gonna sit at this special table down front and start the booing and all, but you know how they always say adequate rest is a must with viruses."

Is this what I've been campaigning for? This end of carefreeness?

"Tomorrow's Saturday, Peg. You can sleep in. Being up late one night isn't going to kill you." I cannot bear this reversal of roles.

*   *   *   *   *

I am closeted in the guest room upstairs trying to write when I hear Joe come in the front door.

"Hi, Peg."

"Whadaya want?"

"I got the car filled up. I had them check the tires, too. It's all ready for you tonight."

"Okay, okay," grunts Peg, as much as to say, Will you stop bothering me. She bangs upstairs and barges into the guest room.

"You are terrible to your father, Peggie. Why do you treat him like that?"

"I know I'm terrible to both you guys, but it's the only way you'll leave me alone. I mean, if you guys come in and I say 'Hi' like 'I'm glad to see you,' you attach yourselves to me."

"Are your tactics working?"

"Well, lately I've been wonderin' if they're not backfiring in the long run. Like the more I act like I don't like you, the more you try to make me like you. But in the short run they're very effective. Like right now you're sitting there wanting to write, but as long as you're nice to me, I'm gonna stay here bothering you."

"You're bugging me to death, Margaret Woodson. You know I'm trying to write. Out. Now."

Peg slinks toward the door. "There, you see, I'm leaving. You hurt my feelings, but I'm leaving. It's the only way with you and father that works."

Later when Joe and I come back from a weekend out of town, I ask Peg how we can best prepare her for life on her own. "Go out of town for three days, mother." Get out of my life forever, mother. Everything she says to me these days she says against the crescendo of that drum roll.

"When are you guys gonna start acting your age? All I ask is that you *leave me alone.*"

Peggie does not want to be questioned; I can handle that. Peggie does not want to be controlled; I can handle that. Peggie does not want to be close; that I cannot handle. I keep getting sick. I, who have hardly been sick in my life, get one cold after another and endless sore throats. And I cry a lot.

Joe is only home one or two nights a week, and he values these family times highly. "Can't you ask John to call back after 'Laverne and Shirley'?" he asks.

"Whatever we have to do, just let's get it over with." Only Peg's body remains in the room with us. "Can I go *now?*" she sneers the minute the last "schemele schmazle" fades.

How we pressure Peg, consciously or subconsciously, to *stand by us*—by tension, by tears, by treating her to a full tank of gas. If I so much as say I'm going to miss her when she's gone, she beats her drums of rebellion fortissimo.

"I'm not saying it to keep you here, Peggie. Your father and I know we've held you too tightly. We'd encourage you to go even if you didn't want to."

"Really? Boy, that's a relief. I gotta admit, you guys do a lot better than some of my friends' parents."

Only when we sign the surrender papers do the war drums stop drumming.

* * * * *

Peg arranges a reunion of her Mohican cabin mates. Spring has risen among us, and with the daffodils comes Peg's dream of conquering the Mohican mountain. Joe and I make our annual two-day pilgrimage to the lodge at Mohican State Park, and Peg agrees to come with us with the understanding that when Glad and Betty appear on the second day, she will disappear with them never to be seen by us again.

On the first day she takes Joe and me to see her mountain. I decide to climb a bit of it, but it has rained the day before, and I feel like I'm suctioning my way up a steep wall of barely congealed mud gelatin. I make it just a few yards up before I slide and fall and roll back down through the ooze. My London Fog, my newly set hair, all of me drips muck.

Well, good. I'm glad I couldn't climb Peggie's mountain. I've mountains of my own to climb. How would she feel if she couldn't climb her mountain and I could? How would she feel if she could climb her mountain and her mother could, too?

"I climbed the mountain," she announces as she struts into the house the next night. "It wasn't even very hard. I just went slowly and kept stopping to rest, and I had a thick branch I used as a staff, and Betty and Glad kept spurring me on.

"The only thing was when we got to the top, nothing was there—just another mountain. Betty wanted to know if I expected bugles blowing. I don't know what I expected, but it was anti-climactic."

"Why was it important for you to make it to the top, Peg?"

"I didn't want to be the only one in the class who couldn't do it. Do you always quit if you can't do something the first time you try? My goodness, mother. Especially if you should have been able to do it, and you're pretty sure you could the next time? What kind of question is that to ask?"

Peg runs upstairs, rummages through the 12th grade folder in her file cabinet, and comes back to throw a piece of notepaper at me. "I've been knowing I was going to climb the mountain for five months, mother." The paper is dated 10/10 and has just one sentence on it.

I AM GOING TO CLIMB THE MOHICAN MOUNTAIN!

Eighteen Years Old

I don't like beer. I don't want to go to R movies. And I don't have anybody to elope with. So what's the point of being eighteen, mother?" In the end, though, Peg decides that a good point to begin eighteen would be tickets to a John Denver concert at the Coliseum—ten-dollar tickets, nothing less.

The day the tickets go on sale, Joe waits outside the May Co., where the ticketron is located, before the store opens. An employee lectures the group about not running through the store and then lifts the gate. Joe is underneath and halfway across the store before the man has the gate all the way up. Fans stream to the escalator from every entrance, up the escalator, and across the second floor.

"I don't want to brag," Joe tells Peg, "but I have to say that not many people got to the ticketron before I did."

"Ya know, mother," Peg tells me, "we gotta have a chapter in this new book you're writing about what a nice father father is. Did I tell you I already decided what I'm getting him for his birthday? A little 45 record called 'They Don't Make Them Like My Daddy Anymore.' I know it will make him happy.

"Remember how when we used to play Probe, and I'd write father *Fat-her* on the score pad, and father didn't like it? Didn't we have fun with him over that? I wonder if he'd catch on if I just called him *phonetic father.*"

Peg washes her hair every morning, but on the big day she washes it again in the afternoon. Gladie goes to the concert with us. I go just to be with Peg on her birthday celebration, but before the concert is over, I am screaming along with the best of them, clapping and stomping to "Grandma's Feather Bed."

It takes an hour and a half to get out of the parking lot, but Joe does not get tense.

"Ya know, Glad," I hear Peg say in the back seat, "I'm really proud of my father the way he's letting me grow up. Can you believe he actually told me it would be up to me when and if I had therapy? And he hasn't gone back on it either.

"Did you know I visited the library at junior high the other day, Gladie? They had my book! Mrs. Murphy says they can't keep it on the shelf. I mean, all kinds of kids are taking out my book!" I can tell from the pride in her voice how much it means to Peg to finally achieve popularity with all kinds of kids in junior high.

So how come she didn't tell me about the book? Why Gladie and not me? Then I remember a remark she made a few weeks ago. "You do realize, mother, that this second book you're writing about me will be the last one you'll be able to write about me? I mean, I don't talk to you about things any more. I talk to other people now."

I feel myself *contracting* in the front seat of the car.

"I asked Mrs. Murphy about Eugene, Gladie, and she said he was away in a correctional school. I sure hope he turns out all right. Have you noticed that I don't get made fun of at school any more? The only thing I still feel bad about is that I'm mostly the one asking other kids to do things, and I never know if they really want to.

"Do I look eighteen, Gladie?"

* * * * *

Are you aware, mother, that I still don't know for absolutely sure where I'm going to college? Why can't there be one college with a nice campus, a good English department, and lots of financial aid? I don't know what to do. And each school is so different in the way it thinks that whichever one I go to, I'm going to come out a different person.

"I mean, I want to have a good time, but then again I do want to learn stuff. I think I'll go to Huss," she says, referring to a third college she has visited, one that stresses academic excellence. "I never had so much fun in my life as when I went to Patterson, but that's all it was mostly. I'd get tired of it.

"I do like being at the top of my class, though. What if at Huss most of the kids are on top of me? I didn't do too hot on my SATs, you know."

"Maybe you have an innate wisdom that doesn't compute, Peg."

"Yeah, but what about those tests I took a couple years ago that said I had outstanding manual dexterity and should work on an assembly line? That I couldn't be a writer because I didn't have high enough general learning ability? That was funny about those test scores getting lost, wasn't it, mother?"

Not so funny, Peg, when you consider that your counselor and I agreed that the best thing that could happen to those test scores was that they stay lost.

I tell Peg about how C. S. Lewis couldn't get into Oxford because he failed their exam in elementary math. He finally got exempt because of the war. He said it was a good thing because at no time in his life would he have been able to pass that exam in elementary math.

"Good old brilliant, logical C. S. Lewis," crows Peg. "I bet he wouldn't have scored high in general learning ability either."

She spends days filling out applications, giving up on one college whose admission procedures are so tedious she decides she doesn't want to go anyplace "that would put you through all that before they even get you." She writes an essay on her personal Christian growth for another college.

I have grown up in a Christian home. Both of my parents are devout Christians and are well-versed in the Bible. They have always been willing to help me with any questions I might have. My church has also helped me grow. Presently I have my own Sunday School class of first and second graders and learn through teaching them. In church my father's sermons are interesting and thought-provoking. I also enjoy our youth group. We have a closely knit group and grow together. Another influence has been my friends. They are of a high caliber, and we encourage each other. My Christian growth has been affected by all of these factors.

"Of course, I know the most important thing is that wherever I go, I end up a better Christian, but even there it's not easy. Why can't there be one college where you think about God and feel God close at the same time?

"Have you noticed how tired I've been lately, mother? I mean, I am really tired all the time, and I keep not being able to catch my breath. I never had that happen to me before."

I look at Peg sitting quietly at the kitchen table panting as though she just ran around the block, and fear hits me like a migraine when I haven't had one for a long time—a unique, I-can't-stand-it pain that makes me sick all over, and worse for its absence and worse for the memory of it.

"Now don't go getting ideas about my not going away to college, mother. I'm going no matter what. But why won't God tell me where to go? I'll go wherever He wants if He'll only tell me . . . write it in the sky. . . .

"I'm going to Huss! Huss, here I come! I've definitely made up my mind! Do you think I should go to Huss?"

*　*　*　*　*

Remember that part of *If I Die at Thirty* where we went upstairs to rock in my room?" Peg asks. "And you said, 'In our family we touch a lot.' Well, we don't touch at all in our family any more, do we?"

"We surely don't, Peg. Your father and I saw a bumper sticker the other day that said, *Have you hugged your kid today?* Daddy laughed and said somebody should make a sticker that says, *Has your kid let you hug her today?*"

"You don't think I'm weird, do you, not wanting to be kissed or anything? On 'Eight Is Enough' those kids are always hugging their father."

I suggest that maybe her new reserve with her father and me has something to do with her looking on her body more and more as a sexual thing, that perhaps it doesn't seem right to her to kiss and hug people for whom she doesn't have sexual feelings. "I don't know, Peg. Do you have a theory?"

"Sometimes I think the sex thing has spread out somehow."

"Maybe you feel like we're owning you when we put our arms around you, Peg, and your not wanting to be hugged is your way of saying, 'I'm cutting loose from you guys.'"

I assure Peg that she isn't alone in feeling as she does. That one friend tells me that when she was Peggie's age, every time her father kissed her on the cheek, she thought, *How gross.* And another friend never was able to sit between her parents in the car without feeling smothered.

"In all her talking about it," I tell Joe in bed, "she never hints that the reason she doesn't act like she loves us is that she doesn't love us." The theorizing doesn't help much, though, for despite my understanding talks with Peg, I have less and less feeling that she does love me. I have to reason it out, and brain cells are not made of stuff the knowledge of love can pass through.

"I have the sense that you love me," I tell Joe.

"I sure am glad."

"Do you have the sense that I love you?"

"I sure do," mumbles Joe, turning over so I can scratch the back of his neck.

I don't require emotional displays; the simplest affirmation will do.

If I forget myself with Peggie, though, and put my hand on her shoulder, she jumps back as though I've burned her. "Don't touch the kid," she moans. If I say, "I love you," she says, "Okay, okay," which being interpreted reads, "Must you, mother?"

The distance Peg puts between herself and me devastates me, but I give her the freedom to put the distance there. Joe, on the other hand, cannot tolerate the sterile atmosphere she imposes on us and from which she will leave us. "I know you don't want me to do this," he says when he goes off for any length of time, "but I'm going to do it anyway." And he kisses the top of her head.

Peg hangs her head; with Joe she endures. But in her heart, the more he insists, the more she resists. "She can't truly say yes to us, Joe," I tell him, "unless we let her first say no."

* * * * *

I am sick again, in bed with chills and fever, and covered with a rash. The doctor says it's a virus so rare it as yet has no name. I am sick of being sick.

I attended a seminar on grief recently. The leader said that when a sad thing happens to you, it produces a tension in your spirit and consequently in your body. When you cry, when you release the tension in your spirit, your body also returns to normal. If, however, you repress your tears, the tension in your body mounts. All the body's systems are thrown out of kilter, but the first system to go is your immunological system. Thus, people who live with unresolved grief are often sick.

I lie in bed now shaking and itching, and I know I need professional help. Being in no condition to go get it, I conjure up a psychiatrist in my mind. She pulls up the rocking chair and sits down beside me.

"I don't think the grief I can't resolve has to do with death," I tell her. "I think about Joey dying, and I cry, and I feel better. I think about Peggie dying, and I cry, and I feel better. It's when I think about Peggie going away to college that I can't cry."

"Can you think of any factor involved in Peggie's going away to college that would not be involved in her dying?" asks the psychiatrist.

For a question like this I need professional help?

The psychiatrist just rocks and waits for my answer.

"The only thing I can think of," I say when the silence becomes too oppressive, "is that if Peg died, her going would be involuntary. But with college, she just keeps saying that she can't wait to get out of here. I've given her the best I have for eighteen years, and all she feels is this mania to get away from me."

Suddenly I cry, and I cannot stop crying, great convulsive sobs. "I guess that must be it," I tell the woman beside my bed.

She explains that it is not sadness itself, but the intensifiers of sadness that loom so large in our hearts that we cannot cry over them because we dare not admit to them. Complicating my sadness, she says, are the rejection I feel at Peggie's eagerness to leave and my anger at her for the rejection.

It might help me, she adds, to realize that some daughters reject their mothers on a conscious level just because they feel so reliant on them, so admiring of them on a subconscious level. I cannot believe that Peg admires me on any level, but the doctor insists that often it is the young people who love their parents most who have to work up the biggest head of hate to chug away from them.

"Peggie has no idea of the effect she's having on you, Mrs. Woodson. Adolescents insult everything about their parents, with the most inventive cruelty, for years on end. But then they're insulted if we hint that they've hurt our feelings."

Then the nice doctor tells me she's afraid our time is up, just like Bob Newhart always told his patients on TV.

I thank her and tell her she is a good therapist and cheap, and then I cry some more. And then I yell for Peggie.

"I found out why I'm sick all the time," I tell her, my sobs and chills synchronized into one gigantic heaving process.

"Now wait a minute. You're not gonna make me feel guilty for you being sick."

I tell Peggie about grief intensifiers and immunological systems and that she jolly well better feel responsible for my being sick because she jolly well is responsible. I also tell her it is a sign of childhood always to insist that nothing is your fault.

"It's all my fault, then? Is that what you want me to believe, that every time you get sick it's all my fault? Well, I don't believe it! And how do you think I feel anyway with you getting sick every time we think about college? I can't go off and leave you on your deathbed." She sits on the floor inside the door of my room, too tired from her own illness to stand and afraid to get any closer to me for fear of catching mine.

I tell Peg that my impaired self-image is my own responsibility, that her behavior wouldn't make me sick if I weren't overly sensitive to rejection. But since I am, she is jolly well right when she says she is in a tight spot, and she jolly well better realize that it is to her advantage as well as mine that we work things out.

I reach down to scratch my feet. Why is my head pounding like this?

"Well, whadaya want me to do? Just what exactly? I don't even know what I've done wrong."

"Well, for starters you don't have to say *yuk* with so much gusto if I accidentally brush up against you."

"I'm kidding when I do that."

"No, you're not kidding, Peggie. And you weren't kidding that time you were sitting on the stairs telling me how much you were going to miss your friends when you went away and how much you weren't going to miss me."

"I never said that."

"Oh, yes you did. You said it deliberately, and you enjoyed saying it, and you're always telling me how dumb I am."

"Yeah, so dumb you write books."

"Remember the other day when you said that by the time you get to college you won't be able to talk to me about anything, because I won't know anything you know to talk about?"

"Well, you are dumb, mother. There's an awful lot of stuff you don't know."

"There, now how do you think that makes me feel? You're so kind to your friends. I don't care what anybody says. I don't believe you don't know it when you're cruel to me."

Peg sits in the door of my sickroom and glares at me in silence. And I, on my side, have blown my anger out. There is just one more question I must ask.

"Will you miss me at all when you leave, Peg?"

"There's only one reason I want to get out of here, mother, and that's so I can do what I want to do. Of course I'll miss you mother." But she smiles that little secret smile of hers as she says it, the little smirk that says, Little do you know, mother.

Oh, Peggie.

I want to ask, Peggie, do you love me at all? But I am not brave enough for that.

* * * * *

*F*ollowing *Joey Home* has just been published, and a Family Bookstore gives an autograph party for Peggie and me in honor of both Joey's book and hers. Peggie wears a new blue dress, and we are honored with corsages, and door prizes are given away every hour, and Peggie works hard at keeping calm.

"Now, for goodness sakes, let's preserve our mother-daughter image," I whisper.

"Nothing doing, mother," this daughter whispers back. "We have to be real if we want anybody to believe us."

Well, Peg's real with me all right.

Before we left the house today, I made reservations for our summer vacation and asked Peg if she wanted to come with us this year. I was sure she wouldn't, but didn't want to exclude her without asking.

"What?" she shrieked, her voice rising to treble heights of incredulity. "Me go on vacation with you guys?"

Peg can be all too real with me for my liking.

But then, evidently remembering our psychiatrist-provoked confrontation of a few days earlier, she added, "What I mean to say, mother, is that much as I would adore to go to the Adirondacks with you and father, I am afraid I have already finalized my summer plans and will have to forego the pleasure."

Well, I give up! Is it so much to ask that Peggie be both Peggie and polite?

The Family Bookstore is near our optometrist, and when the autograph party is over, I ask Peggie to go with me to pick out a pair of glasses.

"Do I have to? I was going to spend the afternoon with Betty." She comes reluctantly.

I try on all the frames the optometrist's wife can find for me, but none will do. Finally the optometrist takes over. "All right," he asks in his thick German accent, "do you joost vant glasses, or do you vant smart?"

"Smart," Peg answers. "She vants smart."

"Oh, honey, look! They're perfect!" I exclaim over the first pair of glasses the optometrist suggests. "But they're way out of my price range."

"You have to get them, mother. You can pay for them with my graduation money."

"Oh, Peggie. I couldn't take your graduation money."

"Well, my college money then. Everything extra around here goes into my college fund. How do you think that makes me feel? You ought to have something special once in a while."

"All right, if you want me to, I'll pay for part of them out of our college money."

As the tears cascade down Peggie's cheeks, I think of how we have sacrificed to buy her glasses through the years—the wire-rims in the eighth grade and the pink and blue shell frames for her senior picture—and I realize that too much love has bonded us for too long for Peg to walk away and never come back. Her antagonism toward me is genuine, but so is her affection.

I know that at the very least I will always be Peg's roots. A safe place for her to come to when the storms are fiercest; a warm, welcome place for her to come for celebrations of joy; even perhaps, God willing and Peggie willing, a home encircled by hedges for her to come to for many summer vacations with her own children. Prickly hedges, perhaps, but real.

Oh, I know Peggie has a lot more walking away to do before she can walk back to me, but every time I wear my new, outsized glasses with the frosted beige designer frames, I see a bit more clearly that that day will come.

*   *   *   *   *

May and June are happy-scary, bittersweet months for Peggie. Momentous, milestone happenings just keep happening, but all the while Peg knows not that the end is coming, but that the end is upon her.

First she wins a three-hundred-dollar scholarship from the Suburban West PTA, and then a two-hundred-dollar scholarship from the Kiwanis Club of which her father is a member. She investigates and decides she did not get the money because of her father. "I'll keep it then," she decrees.

Maxi, the genius, says that Peggie is more likely to get scholarships than she is, because the people who give scholarships prefer overachievers to those with natural brilliance. "Can you believe she actually said that, mother—even if it's true?"

Peg will have a hard time working in college with her therapy and aerosols taking twenty hours a week, and Joe and I encourage her to put her scholarship money in a special account from which she can draw for her personal living expenses. "So you won't have to keep holding your hand out to us, Peg."

"But I'm not ready to be on my own. I don't know how to budget. I don't know how to do income tax. I don't know how to get insurance on a car."

On Recognition Night most of Peg's friends are honored for academic achievement. Peg gets two trophies, one for a four-point average and the other for excellence in English—her most earnest wish come true. Peggie wins the English award! Joe and New York grandmother both parade down front and take pictures of her shaking hands with the presenter.

"John's parents just had a what-are-you-going-to-do-with-your-life talk with him," Peg tells me later. "He's too beat to move." John, it seems, has always wanted to be a composer, but now he has to face the fact that it isn't easy to make a living as a composer. He thinks he'll sell real estate.

"And he's so talented, mother. I've already told him that if I ever should get married, I'm going to use this piece he and Maxi wrote instead of the Wedding March. Do you have any idea how hard it is watching your friends watch their dreams die?"

As graduation day grows closer, the signing of yearbooks becomes more pleasurable and more poignant. Peggie has a record of what people write in her yearbook, of course, but in her 12th grade folder she also has a record of what she writes in theirs.

John won't sign Peg's book until everyone else has, because he wants to write something no one else will see. "I suppose you want to read it, mother."

"Do you want me to?"

"I think I'll keep it to myself for a while."

As graduation day arrives, Peg gives me a list of all the smiley face items she has accumulated during her school years to preserve for all time in our memory box.

> sticky blue fuzzy
> rain hat
> playing cards (from Aunt Kate and Uncle Jim)
> typewriter key
> plant pot (I made it)
> used wrapping paper (2 kinds)
> piñata (Derrick made it)
> pads (Mellaril)
> necklaces (3, but for kids)
> frisbee
> mugs (5)
> night light (Smile, God loves you)

And on and on the list goes, fifty-two items in all. Then before I can file it away, Peg draws a border of smile faces around the list, but with their smile lines jagged. "Can you see they're about to crack, mother?"

I have mixed feelings about graduation myself. Peg is one of 750 black specks down there. Then, too, ever since Joey's sixth grade graduation just before his death, I associate such ceremonies with death. I sit there, surrounded by applauding parents, thinking that God is going to let Peggie die fat and happy and on the way up—that she is going to keep on going straight up to God's happy, holy land of everlasting learners.

We have a party for Peg after graduation with a few of our

best friends. Peggie keeps getting called to the phone, and when our guests leave around midnight, new guests arrive. "Me and my friends," says Peg, "we're having our own party."

Then she looks at me apologetically. "My friends and I, right, mother?" But then some need I cannot identify outweighs her need for good grammar, and she says, "No, me and my friends. You got that, mother? Me and my friends are having our own party."

Well, her and her friends sprawl in the family room and mostly look at each other. They are zonked, but they cannot bear not to be together tonight, all but one of them having been together since ninth grade advanced English. They talk about all the parties they have had in our house over the years. John reclines in our big black chair and covers his face with a book. Every once in a while he reaches up and turns a page.

* * * * *

$\mathbf{I}$ can't get used to there being so much of me," Peg wonders aloud, scrutinizing herself sideways in the dressing room mirror. "There must be a foot of me front to back. I can't adjust to so much person."

She turns front on and paints herself onto the glass canvas, inch by inch, with a master's critical eye. Then the self-portrait stirs uneasily and explodes into indignant life. "Just look at that fat. Would you believe it? Shopping for clothes is so demoralizing when my stomach sticks out this way. Now would it not be logical to assume, mother, that if your fat wrinkles, there's too much of it?"

"Maybe you should shop for a girdle, Peg."

"A what—a what?" she stutters, but then gyrates into several infinitesimal stretch contraptions. "Ouch! Oooh! Ow!" she howls. "Boy, I'll tell you one thing, mother. When you're trying on a girdle, never let go half-way up!"

Dressing rooms bring out the giggles in Peggie and me, but not for long this time, as Peg's stomach sticks out even with a girdle, and that is no giggling matter. C.F.ers often have stomachs that protrude somewhat, and Peg's has always been a concern to her. Now she is sure that most of her recently gained pounds have settled in her middle parts, and her stomach is a weighty embarrassment.

A while ago she made us all sit up with her and watch the film *Just a Little Inconvenience,* the story of a man who had lost both an arm and a leg. At the end of the movie, he skis down a difficult slope, and a friend says, "Not bad for a man with a handicap." The young hero replies, "What do you mean *handicap?* This is just a little inconvenience."

Peg worried all through the movie that he wouldn't actually say the words. "Isn't that magnificent?" she warbled when finally he did.

So when she is carrying on in Penney's dressing room about every pair of pants she tries on making her stomach more noticeable, I poke her paunch playfully and say, "Oh, it's just a little inconvenience."

"That's how much you understand, mother. That's the one

thing the kids still laugh about—clothes and how you look—even my friends. And who knows what it will be like at college? Me having C.F. is a little inconvenience, but my stomach sticking out is in an entirely different category."

In the evening as she takes her aerosol, she calls me to listen to a tape on which a male voice sings the words of Jesus, "In the world you shall have tribulation, but be of good cheer. I have overcome the world."

"Isn't that beautiful, mother? I can hardly listen to it without crying. I don't know why, except the vocalist has such a nice, deep voice! I think maybe that's the way Jesus actually sounded when He said those words."

She darts a pained glance down at her belly bulging even inside her new, slenderizing, navy pants. "Like I think *He* understands, mother. Like maybe He's actually saying those words . . . to me."

* * * * *

Early Friday afternoon we deposit Peggie in her dorm room, a colorless, dirty room. I bustle about dusting with a sock, while Peg flops on the bed. "Do you have to make so much noise about it, mother? I'm just here for orientation weekend."

Well, I know, but how will Peg survive even for the weekend shut up in this oven of a room, not knowing a living soul, not letting her mother arrange for someone to do her therapy?

I control myself, however, and when we leave, Peg issues mighty words of praise. "You guys are doing better than I expected. No mush."

Joe and I trudge down the endless hall of faceless doors. "That was a long walk, wasn't it?" Joe asks when finally we reach the lounge.

Well, the past four years have been a long walk—more like a forced march.

I drift in and out of Peg's room at home while she's gone, examining for the first time the border she has tacked up on one side of the room—red, yellow, and green sheets of construction paper on which she has printed her favorite Bible verses.

In conclusion, my brothers, fill your minds with those things that are good and that deserve praise: things that are true, noble, right, pure, lovely, and honorable. Philippians 4:8

We know that in all things God works for good with those who love him. Romans 8:28

My deep desire and hope is that I shall never fail my duty, but that at all times, and especially right now, I shall be full of courage, so that with my whole being I shall bring honor to Christ, whether I live or die. Philippians 1:20

Well, whatever you do, whether you eat or drink, do it all for God's glory. 1 Corinthians 10:21

Every good and perfect gift is from above, coming down from the Father of heavenly lights. James 1:17 For you are all children of the light and of the day, and do not belong to darkness and night. 1 Thessalonians 5:5

In the world you shall have tribulation; but be of good cheer, I have overcome the world. John 16:33

Are they there with her as she's oriented to her future, these treasured guides to her past?

Peg gets a ride home on Monday morning, and Joe and I pounce on her as soon as she's in the house, beside ourselves to hear how things have gone. Peg is not of a mind to talk. Finally Joe and I settle down to read in the family room. Peg follows us and chatters nonstop for one hour, twenty-three minutes, and sixteen seconds by the clock.

"I was pretty bored late Friday night—and hungry, too," she says. "So I went up and down the hall knocking on doors to see if anybody had anything to eat. I got to know quite a few kids that way.

"Like Alice, the girl next-door. I mean, she wants to be a nurse, and she did therapy on me, and she's desperate for the money, and she thinks God put her in the room next to mine so she could do therapy on me, and I think He did, too, and I found her myself, mother.

"Now I probably should tell you guys that just because John Huss is a church school doesn't mean all the kids go to church. I mean, a lot of them were out all Saturday night getting drunk and making out. Like I actually saw some of them weaving down the hall early Sunday morning.

"Now don't go worrying about how the ones who do that stuff are going to influence me, father. I'm the one who intends to influence them.

"The only thing I didn't like was being on the second floor and how tired I got walking from building to building.

"You want to know what I did on Saturday night? Well, it was so hot I thought I would collapse of heat exhaustion if I stayed in my room, and there was this ledge you could crawl out on through this storage room, and I rounded up three other girls, and we took our sleeping bags and slept out there. You can't imagine how peaceful it was under the stars, and so cool.

"But then this night guard found us—and, you guys, we were so scared. But he said he wouldn't report us, and he checked on us with his flashlight all through the night. Then at 5:30 I left my sleeping bag out there and tip-toed inside for therapy, and when the night guard came back, he could only see three mounds on the ledge, and he was looking in the bushes all underneath for my body, and he was telling the story all over campus.

"When we left, some of the kids told me they were glad I was coming to Huss, that I really livened things up."

Peg spends the rest of the day talking to Glad and John and Betty on the phone. In more ways than I expected, though, she also spends the day with Joe and me. "It's pretty good to be home," she says. "Boy, my own room. It looks pretty good, my own room. You guys won't change a lot of things while I'm gone, will you? I mean, what if I come back and the spider plant has babies?"

* * * * *

Two C.F. patients die during the two weeks Peggie is in the hospital—a young minister and Jamie, a friend of Peg's for many years.

"It took me three days to get up my nerve to go in and talk to Jamie," Peg tells me on my first visit. "But I remembered how you said that when Joey was dying, nobody went near him, and a dying person was still a living person, so I finally went in.

"The first thing he said to me was, 'I can't seem to get off this oxygen.' I could tell he was scared. I've been going in there every day. Even if they have the door closed, I ask the nurse if I can just go in and say hi.

"When Jamie's feeling better, he talks to me about how he's going to finish high school a year late and all." Peg buries her face in her hands and bawls. "It wouldn't be so bad if he weren't so scared.

"I haven't watched 'All My Children' in five days, mother. I'm having withdrawal symptoms. I mean, two days I went down and shut myself in this kid's room who doesn't have a TV, and two days I gave the kid my TV, and the fifth day I took a nap. It's not easy, let me tell you. Do you realize I will never know what happens to Philip and Chuck and Donna and everybody?"

"Why are you giving it up, Peg?"

"It doesn't fit my favorite verses.

"You know how I'm going to decorate my room at Huss if smiley faces are considered old-fashioned? With bubbles! Bubbles with wise sayings inside them!

"Did you know I sneaked into the shower room the other day and hid Laurel's clothes while she was behind the curtain? Well, she came flying into my room wrapped in a towel, screaming for my robe. Then she said she didn't know what she would do without me and wait till she got her hands on those boys down the hall. Laurel hasn't been in with me much before."

Peg says that she does not want me to visit her more than once a week, especially when she's too tired to go out of the hospital to eat. That she doesn't know what to do with me when I come oftener than that. Well, talk my ear off is what she does with me. And give me her dirty clothes to wash.

Some of the older patients, she says, don't even tell their parents when they're in the hospital. They don't want to go back to being kids again with their folks fussing over them. "You know how some people get married so they'll have someone to grow old with, mother? Well, lately I've been thinking I might like to get married so I'd have someone to die with.

"I asked Jamie didn't he mind his mother being here so much, but he said, 'No, me and my mom and dad, we're pretty close.'

"I'm getting reinforced for going off to school with so many friends here. We talk about life and death and stuff so much, sometimes I think the world in here is more the real world than the world outside. When the minister died the other night, all the kids came in my room to watch them wheel his body down the hall."

In the middle of the second week, Peg calls at seven o'clock in the morning to tell me Jamie died that night. Never learning, I tear over to the hospital to be with her in her hour of need.

"What on earth are you doing here at this hour?" Peg scoffs. "They put Jamie in a wheelchair yesterday and wheeled him all over the floor. Everybody had a chance to say hi. Wasn't that nice that he got to say hi to everybody? The whole floor's upset today. I mean, some of the kids are crying, and some of them are mad. I'm glad I was in when he died. I'm glad I could visit him.

"I liked that book, The Singer, you gave me the day I checked in, mother. It's hard to read, but it gives me helpful insights. I knew I'd like it as soon as I read the first page.

> For most who live,
> hell is never knowing
> who they are.

"You remember that girl at school who wrote on the back of my senior picture, *I wish I had your peace.* Well, I asked her what she meant, and she said I seemed so self-assured, and I said I wasn't at all self-assured, and she said I knew who I was. But if I do know it, I don't know I know it. Is that because I've always known it?"

I drive home from the hospital in the noonday light. I remember another drive home from the hospital, in the dark, more than four years ago. I remember my pained prayer that the impossible would happen, that *Peggie* would survive. And I pray again; I thank God that she has.

* * * * *

We are taking Peg to Huss forever, or so it seems. Joe removes the back seat from the car to fit all her paraphernalia in—her therapy table, her air compressor, her percussor, the refrigerator for her medications, and the seven-hundred-dollars worth of medications we pray will last till her first visit home at Thanksgiving.

Dr. Rathburn dismissed Peggie from the hospital not knowing what was wrong with her. Her pulmonary function scores were back to what is normal for her, but she was so weak she barely staggered from her room down to the parking garage. "Why can't I catch my breath, mother? I mean, I know you don't know, but what do you think?"

Dr. Rathburn still maintains that it would be better for Peg to give college a try and not make it than for her not to try.

"You know, I keep wondering about this second book you're writing about me, mother," Peg says, squeezed in alongside Joe and me in the front seat of the car. "Like I still think it needs something to liven it up, and you know what would do it? If I died."

"Honestly, Peggie!"

"Well, it would help. Wouldn't you rather read a book about a kid who died than a kid who didn't?"

"You know, Peg, ever since Joey was diagnosed as having cystic fibrosis sixteen years ago, I've had this notion that one of you children might glorify God by dying and one of you might glorify God by living. Now, thus far that is the way it has been, and that is the way I would like to keep it."

"I still want you to give me a week's notice when I'm dying. Remember, you promised? I've got mixed feelings about the whole thing, though. I mean, I'm going to fight when my time comes. There's a lot of stuff I want to do first."

The three of us, with all our normal and abnormal apprehensions, crowded together like this for a six-hour drive, portends interpersonal disaster. Peggie is not helping.

"You remember how unhappy you were with us way back when you were spending all your time in the hospital with Alex and we were afraid you would get too involved?" Joe asks

Peg. "Well, I realized the other day that with all the experience you've had with boys now, I don't worry about that sort of thing any more."

"Really?" squeals Peg.

"And after the decision you made about going to Huss, which I consider a difficult, mature decision, I don't think there's anything I don't trust you about."

"You mean it?"

How much Joe's trust means to Peg. Probably it is the best going-away gift he can give her. And I'm sure her trustworthiness is the finest gift she can give Joe.

"Speaking about trust, father, I don't worry that much about whether I'm going to the right school or not any more. I figure that if God wants me at a certain college, it's because I'll learn certain stuff there. And if I get to the wrong college by mistake, God can still teach me the same stuff one way or another. He can make anything work for good."

Peg is driving now, swaying to the blare of the radio, lilting her usual "Yeah, yeah!" But then she breaks in on the program like a newscaster with a special bulletin that has nothing to do with what precedes or follows it. "Adults, adults! I can't wait to get to college to meet some adults. You guys are ruining this world."

Joe and I have to laugh right out loud.

But we laugh to ourselves that night when Peg is settled in her dorm but casually announces that she thinks she'll spend this last night in the Red Roof Inn with us. In the morning she pulls the covers up over her head and refuses to budge. Only her small, muffled voice emerges.

"I'll probably have the time of my life. Right, mother? Father?"

Right, Peggie.

Epilogue

When Peg came home for Christmas her first year of college, she had such trouble breathing and walking that hospital admissions tried to send her upstairs in a wheelchair.

"I've never—gone up there yet—except on my feet—and I'm not—going up—in a wheelchair now." The words emerged from Peggie's lungs as from a dented, toy foghorn. And indeed she dragged her own way from bench to bench down the long corridors and up to the fourth floor.

Since then, crises with her health, some of them life-threatening, have hospitalized her twice a year or so; but the bad times have been interspersed with good, and Peg has dragged and danced her way through college, till now as this book goes into print, she is preparing to graduate.

She called this past summer from Philadelphia, where she was working as an editorial intern at *Eternity* magazine, to tell me she had just learned that Jenny, her second, best C.F. friend, had died. The girls had grown apart in recent years; still, Jenny's death hit Peg and Joe and me hard. Every C.F. friend mentioned in this book is now dead.

"It can't happen many more times," Peg comforted herself on the phone. "There aren't that many of us left." Then she wrapped her comfort more tightly around herself by counting six friends who could still die and who were, therefore, still alive.

When Peggie first left for college, she wanted to go just far enough away that she could not get home for weekends and we could not get to her. It worked so well that she stayed on in the dorm for the summer after her freshman year and worked nearby. For her sophomore year, however, she transferred to Malone College, a church school in Canton, Ohio, "where the kids are friendlier," and where she has been happy ever since.

The closeness of Malone College to home was incidental but acceptable. "Now that I've established myself, mother, I can come back."

The summer after her sophomore year, Peg chose to live at home and study at the community college—automobile maintenance and karate. "I figure I've been rotten to you guys for half my life," she said, demonstrating a fearsome Tai Kwon Do kick and collapsing on the couch. "I decided to come home for one summer and be nice."

Peg's visits and her phone calls, which she makes in times of ecstasy or stress, not only long-distance but long and collect, leave me feeling whole. Only when I revert to flapping my mother-bird wings in a frenzy of overprotection does Peg revert to her shoo-shoo-get-away-from-me mentality.

Last year on the first day of spring, Peg routed a bunch of kids from their dorm rooms and led a caravan of cars to the base of a hill, on top of which stood a monument, the top of which they decreed to be the highest point in Canton—and from which they stomped and clapped and yawned their welcome to the dawn's early, rosy light.

This year when March 21st rolled around and the kids left their dorms for breakfast, they were transported into an enchanted parking lot: a balloon on which some midnight elf had magic-markered "Happy First Day of Spring" beckoned to them from every antenna of every car.

Peggie continues to celebrate her own parti-colored brand of perennial springtime.

During her junior year, Peg brought home the biggest surprise of her life or mine—a boyfriend. "Can you imagine how good it makes me feel about myself, mother, having been passed over in that department all my life?

"Paul doesn't always feel too good about me, though," she giggled. "I mean, I have explained to him over and over about sex and love and permanent commitment all going together, but he doesn't get it. Now he is really smart, but I finally asked him, 'Do you just not like it, Paul, or do you really not understand?' And he said, 'I really don't understand, Peggie.'

"I hold his hand, that's all. He may not be my boyfriend for a long time, but I bet he'll remember me for a long time."

Peg picks many of her college friends from among the kids involved in drugs and sex. "So many of the pious kids are all alike, father. I get bored around them. Is that awful to say? The kids I hang out with seem more real. I let them know I don't approve of what they do, but I don't preach at them or anything. I'm more like a counselor, and they help me in other ways."

"Are you ever tempted to go your friends' route?" I asked Peg on her most recent visit home.

"I'm tempted not to do things that are right, but I'm not tempted to do the wrong things, because I see how miserable they make everybody. Did you know I talked in sharing chapel the other day, mother? I was scared in front of so many people, but one of my friends told me later I looked cute up there in my bright yellow top kind of bouncing up and down.

"I talked about how everybody could be happy if they'd just make up their minds to get excited about little things. Then I said, 'Now I have a lung disease, and ordinarily I can't climb a flight of stairs without getting out of breath, but right now I can, and it feels so good, I get really happy about it.'

"Then I closed by saying, 'Most people, if they wanted to, could get excited all the time about climbing a flight of stairs without losing their breath.'"

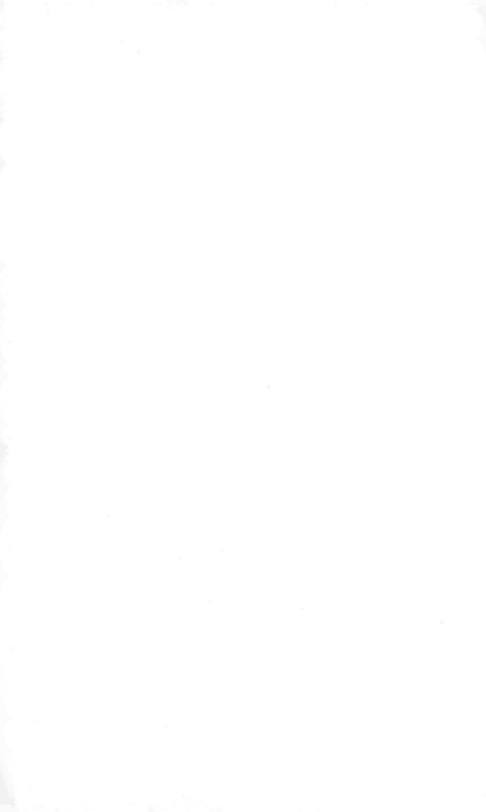